THE HEALTH
OF POPULATIONS

Andrew Harper, MBBS, MPH, DrPH, is a clinical epidemiologist with the Hospital Benefit Fund Occupational Health Services in Perth, Western Australia. Until 1985 he was an associate professor of clinical epidemiology and family medicine at McMaster University. From 1972 to 1976 he was director of community medicine at Royal Prince Alfred Hospital in Sydney. He graduated in medicine from the University of Sydney in 1966 and obtained a doctorate in public health from Harvard University in 1975.

THE HEALTH OF POPULATIONS

AN INTRODUCTION

Andrew C. Harper
MBBS, MPH, DrPH

Springer Publishing Company
New York

To Alex
and Claudia

Copyright © 1986 by Springer Publishing Company, Inc.

All rights reserved

Springer Publishing Company, Inc.
536 Broadway
New York, NY 10012

86 87 88 89 90 / 5 4 3 2 1

Library of Congress Cataloging-in-Publication Data

Harper, Andrew C.
  The health of populations.

  Bibliography: p.
  Includes index.
  1. Public health. 2. Medicine, Preventive.
I. Title.
RA425.H298 1986   362.1   86-21946
ISBN 0-8261-5510-3

Printed in the United States of America

Contents

Acknowledgments xi

Introduction xiii

CHAPTER 1 A Framework for a Population Perspective 1

Concepts of Health and Population 2
  Health 2
  Population 5
The Scientific Basis of Population Health 6
  Introduction 6
  Measuring the Problem 9
  Understanding the Problem 9
  Solving the Problem 9
  Discussion 10
Population Health in Practice 10
  The Inadequacy of Available Data 10
  The Ethics of Health Decisions 11
  Health Decisions as a Political Process 13
Summary 14

CHAPTER 2 The Problem: A General Perspective on Health 16

Disease 17
  Life Expectancy 17
    Methodology 17
    The Evidence 18
  Mortality 18
    Methodology 19
    The Evidence 21
    Causes of Death 22
  Disease Frequency 25

Disability   28
   Institutionalization   29
   Activity Restriction   30
   Emotional Health   31
   Social Health   33
   The Demographic Dimension to Health   34
   Morbidity in Primary Care Practice   36
Summary   39

**CHAPTER 3 The Problem: The Health of
Specific Populations   41**

The American Elderly   42
   Introduction   42
   Mortality   42
   Morbidity   43
   Discussion   44
Cultural Groups   45
   Black Americans   45
     Discussion   47
   Morbidity among Hispanic Americans   47
     Discussion   48
   The Canadian Native Population   49
     Discussion   50
The Poor in Canada   51
   Introduction   51
   Life Expectancy   52
   Mortality   52
   Morbidity   55
   Discussion   56
Groups with Specific Health Problems   57
   Introduction   57
   The Consequences of Disease   58
Summary   61

**CHAPTER 4 Risks I: Concepts and
Methods   62**

McKeown's Historical Perspective   62
   Causes of Death 1848 to 1971   63
   Causes of Death 1700 to 1848   66
   Framework of Analysis   67

Determinants of Health   72
Risk and Natural History   73
    Definitions   73
    Methods   75
Summary   81

CHAPTER 5   Risks II: Causes of Disease   82

Hereditary Factors   82
Behavior and Life Style   84
    Smoking   84
    Alcohol   87
    Diet   89
    Exercise   90
    Reproductive and Sexual Behavior   91
    Driving Behavior   91
    Social Relationships   92
    Discussion   92
Environmental Factors   92
    Occupational Environment   93
    Pollution   97
    The Man-Made Environment   99
Summary   102

CHAPTER 6   Risks III: Selected Diseases and
Their Causes   104

Cancer   104
    Evidence Concerning the Cause of Cancer   105
        Biological Evidence   105
        Epidemiological Evidence   108
    Avoidable Causes of Cancer   110
        Tobacco   110
        Diet   111
        Alcohol   113
        Food Additives   114
        Reproductive and Sexual Behavior   114
        Occupation   114
        Pollution   114
        Industrial Products   114
        Medicines and Medical Procedures   115
    ⌐ Geophysical Factors   115
        Infection   115
    Discussion   116

Ischemic Heart Disease   116
  Risk Factors   117
    Hypertension   117
    Diabetes Mellitus and Hyperglycemia   117
    Smoking   118
    Diet   118
    Serum Cholesterol   120
    Other Factors   120
    Multiple Risk Factors   121
    Psychosocial Factors   121
    Discussion   122
  Biological Aspects   122
  Summary   125

CHAPTER 7   Solutions I: Reducing the Risk of
            Disease   127

Methods   127
Interventions to Reduce Risk   129
  Reducing the Risk due to Smoking   130
    A Safe Cigarette   130
    Control of Other Etiologic or Protective Factors   131
    Cessation of Smoking   131
    Discussion   135
  Changing Diet and Reducing Serum Cholesterol   135
    Discussion   138
  Multiple Risk Factor Reduction   139
    Discussion   141
  Reducing the Consumption of Alcohol   142
  Promoting Safe Driving Behavior   144
    Driver Education   145
    Mass Media and Seat Belt Usage   145
    Legislation   146
    Discussion   148
  Immunization   148
  Summary   150

CHAPTER 8   Solutions II: The Search for
            Effective Therapy   152

The Search for Effective Therapy   154
  Cancer   154

Cardiovascular Disease   157
  Hypertension   157
  Angina Pectoris and Myocardial Infarction   160
  Discussion   163
Methodology   163
  Screening   164
  Clinical Disagreement   164
  Diagnostic Accuracy   165
Summary   167

CHAPTER 9 Solutions III: The Role of the
                Health Care System:
                Organizational Effectiveness
                and Efficiency   168

Organizational Effectiveness   169
  Introduction   169
  Organizational Structure and Health   169
    Type of Health Service   169
    Specific Aspects of Organization   171
    Some General Aspects of Organization   172
  The Process of Care and Health   173
  Availability and Health   173
  Patient Compliance with Health Care   174
  Discussion   175
Efficiency of Health Care   176
  Introduction   176
  Methods   177
  Efficiency of Personal Health Services   178
  Interpretation   180
Summary   182

CHAPTER 10 Population Health in
                 Perspective   184

Health and Health Care   184
  The Avoidance of Disease   186
  Curing Disease   187
  Reducing Morbidity   187
Science and Health Policy   188
  Identification and Description of Health
    Problems   189

Research into the Origins of Illness, Handicap, and
Disease   190
Research into the Effectiveness and Efficiency of
Interventions   190
The Patient and Health Care   191
A Population Perspective on Health   194

References   199

Index   217

Acknowledgments

This book has resulted from the ideas and interests of many people. In the early 1980s, circumstances at McMaster University favored developments in Population Health. The relevance of a broad perspective on health had been impeccably explained by Thomas McKeown while a visiting professor at McMaster in the late 1970s. McKeown's work had stimulated Fraser Mustard, then Vice-President of Health Sciences, to pursue his interest in the somewhat strained relationship of health and health care. A university-wide forum within which to bring faculty and students together to study Population Health was created by the Graduate Program in Health Care Practice in 1981. Under the innovative leadership of Gina Browne, Fraser Mustard was invited to expand and develop a course on Population Health. He welcomed the opportunity and proceeded to attract collaboration from a wide range of diciplines including Nursing, Clinical Epidemiology and Biostatistics, Philosophy, Pathology, Family Medicine, Psychiatry, Geography, Business Administration, and Internal Medicine. It was his suggestion that this book be written. Financial assistance was provided by a teaching and learning grant from the University as well as considerable support from the Faculty of Health Sciences and the Department of Clinical Epidemiology and Biostatistics. The ongoing interest and backing from Peter Tugwell, Chairman of Clinical Epidemiology and Biostatistics, has been essential to the completion of the project. This support included typing the manuscript, which was done by Lorna Bingham. Over the two years of preparing the manuscript, Lorna's energy, her friendly manner, her proficiency and willingness to work hard have been of the greatest help to me.

A lot of the stimulus for this text came from graduate students in Health Care Practice, Business Administration, and Design Measurement and Evaluation. Their refreshing and practical ideas were of great value.

Behind all of the above has been the continual support of my wife Dorothy. Not only has she helped me through version after version and provided the encouragement to keep writing, but her ideas and experience have enriched and broadened my approach to the subject. Finally, I want to acknowledge that the advice and friendship of David J. C. Read and the support of Margot Harper over many years have allowed my particular interest in medicine to be brought together in this publication.

Despite the help of others I must take responsibility for what has been included and omitted.

ANDREW HARPER
Hamilton, Ontario
1985

Introduction

The community-wide perspective of public health practice and the individual orientation of clinical medicine have been separate and distinct for most of this century. In recent years, interest has developed in integrating these two approaches within a unified population perspective on health (Lipkin & Lybrand, 1982). This integrated view has developed in response to accumulating evidence that present methods of medical practice are achieving only modest and limited improvements in the population's health.

My interest in the importance of taking both a specific and general view of the patient was firmly established when I was an emergency room resident in the children's hospital in Sydney. One evening a mother presented with two of her children, both of whom had mild asthma. The asthma itself was uncomplicated and required no more than the medication which had already been prescribed by both the local doctor and a community hospital physician. Why, then, had this woman traveled 30 miles by public transport to have her children seen? On inquiry, the mother was very anxious about her children's asthma and appeared to have a limited understanding of the disease. It was as though little had been explained to her. However, on further inquiry she revealed that her husband had died from asthma that had been described initially as being mild and not serious. Complicating her justifiable fears were other factors. Since her husband's death she had worked operating a manual laundry press. In recent months this gave her chest pain, but not having been given time off work, she had not received help for this. To add to her responsibilities, her eldest daughter, still in high school, had recently added her own baby to the household of six children. She felt trapped by her situation and could foresee no prospect of relief. She had been unable to find the support she needed from the medical profession, her employer, or her community. There was no simple solution to this woman's predicament at the time, but neither is there a solution today. The problems of low income, possible heart disease, a large family to support, social isolation, and her own personal needs and fears required a more comprehensive approach to health care than is routinely available. Training that is limited to the treatment of disease fails to prepare health professionals for the many and varied problems they will face in practice.

The majority of diseases today have a chronic course protracted over many years. The disease itself is often only part of the patient's problem, and the adverse effects of illness on the quality of life are the cause of much suffering and disability. While medical treatment is focused on physical problems, it is common for a patient's fears and apprehension to go unattended. In addition, there is a preoccupation in our health care system with waiting for disease to occur rather than preventing it. We know that cigarettes, alcohol, overeating, driving automobiles, and unprotected work places are all causes of disease and disability. Another problem of the affluent society is that the benefits of affluence are not equally distributed and many groups within society are underprivileged, underserviced, and experience more illness than the middle class majority. It may be that the extravagances of unnecessary investigations and expensive, unproven treatments divert money and effort from useful strategies as yet untried.

The fallacy of the 20th century approach to health may be as extreme as was proposed in the 1980 Reith Lectures (Kennedy, 1980). Society may have hitched its wagon to the wrong star, scientific medicine. Science, Kennedy argues, has destroyed our faith in religion and challenged our trust in magic. In treating illness the scientific method is portrayed as the appropriate method, whereas skills in resolving guilt, fear, depression, conflict, or misunderstanding may also be important. The child dying of leukemia is both a scientific problem and a complex emotional, spiritual, and social problem. At the very least we need to critique and review the manner in which disease and illness are managed today. The solution will hopefully be some combination of the present system, with new and effective measures to address the outstanding problems and deficiencies.

The Health of Populations is an attempt at developing a systematic and factual basis for a more complete, unified, and sensitive approach to health than exists at present. I do not feel that the responsibility for health should rest exclusively with health professionals. I suspect that the health system would be more responsive and cognizant of health needs once patients and the public make themselves more informed of health issues and take an active and energetic part in defining health priorities.

Population health is the study of the health of whole communities and groups. Its major aim is to find ways to reduce illness and handicap among populations at high risk. Populations at an increased risk of health problems include the poor, the elderly, the disabled, ethnic groups, the young, the affluent, occupational groups, and those already afflicted with disease. Policy decisions that influence the health of these groups are being made every day, but the effectiveness of these decisions is hindered by our lack of knowledge or failure to use available evidence. The scientific basis of health policies would be greatly improved if more legislators, administrators, health professionals, and members of the public had a thorough understanding of which sectors of society are at a high risk of illness, of the causes of the major disabilities and diseases, and of the measures which are successful in improving health.

Population health is not a discrete domain of medical practice. Due to its comprehensive perspective it encompasses and overlaps many fields. Community medicine, public health, biostatistics, and epidemiology are core disciplines of population health. Clinical disciplines such as family medicine, occupational health, the therapies, nursing, clinical psychology, social work, pediatrics, obstetrics, psychiatry, internal medicine, geriatrics, and numerous other specialties all play important parts in and contribute to our understanding of population health. Social sciences including health economics, medical sociology, social psychology, and medical anthropology strive to explain the behavioral dimension to population health.

The relevance of a population perspective on health stems from a number of factors. Specialization has led to medical treatment being focused on progressively more specific aspects of disease. While specialization has led to notable achievements, from which all society stands to gain, this has made the prescription of medical management for a patient's overall welfare and comfort an increasingly complex task. Biomedical interests tend to overshadow the other aspects of medical care. The growing fragmentation and diversification of medical services emphasize the need for society to keep informed of the patient's general welfare. There is a risk that the quality of life will be jeopardized as medical practice narrows its focus on progressively smaller components of the patient's illness. Accountability is also a major problem. Large sums of money are spent on treatments that have not been evaluated or shown to make a positive contribution to health. Research funds are unequally distributed among the biological and behavioral aspects of illness. The potential gains from national strategies to prevent illness and injury are little publicized, and prevention is a small part of government policy. Primary medical care, where the majority of illness is treated, receives fewer financial incentives, less research money, and less university teaching time than secondary and tertiary medicine. There is an imbalance in the health care system. A broad perspective on health is needed to reduce current biases and to respond more effectively and efficiently to the health needs of society.

An unbiased approach to health policy requires a general understanding of the current state of knowledge of the determinants of illness and disease and of the effectiveness of interventions and modern therapy. It was with this aim in mind that this text has been written. Although a far larger volume is needed to cover the subject completely, I feel that an introduction will prove useful to many readers. *The Health of Populations* is therefore an introductory text on population health. It has been written for students, health care practitioners and policy makers, and individuals wanting an overview of scientific progress. The aims of the book are threefold. The first is to present a selective summary of scientific evidence. The second is to describe the epidemiologic methods needed to appraise the scientific credibility of the evidence. Third, the content has been presented in a format designed to help the reader think of population health problems in a systematic way without being distracted by the vastness of the topic.

The book is organized in the following way. Chapter 1 presents a conceptual framework that provides a way of thinking about population health. Chapters 2 and 3 describe the nature and frequency of the major physical and behavioral health problems of society. To provide consistency to these two chapters, North America has been taken as the principal example, although data from other countries have also been included.

Chapters 4, 5, and 6 are concerned with the cause of disease. In the first of these chapters basic concepts and methods relevant to the risk of disease are presented. McKeown's historical analysis of the determinants of disease is used to demonstrate the importance of human behavior and environment in promoting health, and therefore British data predominate in Chapter 4. The major risk factors and causes of disease are reviewed in Chapter 5, including heredity, smoking, drinking, diet, lack of exercise, sexual behavior, driving, social relationships, the occupational environment, pollution, and the man-made environment. In Chapter 6 the etiology of cancer and heart disease are examined in detail, including both biological and epidemiologic data.

Chapters 7, 8, and 9 are concerned with the effectiveness of preventive and therapeutic interventions and of the health care system itself. Primary prevention is reviewed in Chapter 7, focusing on life-style modification and immunization. Chapter 8 deals with the effectiveness of medical therapy in which cancer, hypertension, and heart disease are used as illustrations. The role of the organization of health services in the effectiveness and efficiency of care is examined in Chapter 9. Data in these chapters are drawn from research conducted in the United States, Britain, Australia, and Canada. The interpretation and implications of a population perspective on health are considered in Chapter 10.

One intention of this book is to add to the reader's appreciation of the importance of referring to original sources of data rather than relying on opinion or other persons' interpretations. Methodological considerations in critiquing scientific evidence are therefore a recurring theme. An effort has been made to reference the text thoroughly and to provide access to original sources of data. Owing to the breadth of topics all data on any given subject could not be included. In the selection of material I have endeavored to be unbiased. The diverse nature of population health has required that in organizing the text emphasis be placed on providing a degree of continuity. The chapters have been organized, therefore, within a simple conceptual framework that is presented in detail in Chapter 1. While each of the subsequent chapters stand alone, for those reading the book in a piecemeal fashion initial reference to this chapter would be helpful.

Chapter 1

A Framework for a
Population Perspective

Health care in the 20th century has been characterized by change involving unprecedented advances in drug therapy, surgical techniques, and investigative methods. The hallmark of these developments has been the creation of vast areas of understanding at the level of diseased organs, cells, and molecules. This disease-oriented era in medical history contrasts with the environmental advances of the public health era which preceded it. During the last century the major advances in health resulted from changes in food supply, sanitation, and water supply, and the death rates from air-, food-, and water-borne infectious diseases fell dramatically. The domain of health endeavor swung like a pendulum from this general environmental focus of the 1800s to a specific biological focus in this century. Medical research today concentrates more than ever before on the physical and biochemical characteristics of disease. *Population health*, as developed in this book, is an integration of the environmental and individual approaches to health and disease.

The purpose of population health is the health of all individuals. Communities are made up of individuals, and in order to do the best for the health of a community each sector must be identified and understood. Health, disease, and illness are so variable that no single approach to their management is sufficient. Health, as an individual and social condition, therefore, needs a comprehensive approach. This comprehensive approach to health should fulfill a number of prerequisites: (1) Health should be defined in terms appropriate to prevailing customs and attitudes. (2) The individuals and groups, whose health is being referred to, need to be identified. (3) A means must exist to measure the actual health state of the community. (4) There should be a practical level of understanding of what is causing health problems. (5)

1

Methods to treat the problems are needed. (6) And finally, an acceptable method for making decisions and policies about health is a prerequisite for making optimal use of the existing information.

CONCEPTS OF HEALTH AND POPULATION

Health

The concept of health is relative to time and circumstances. In the past, when infectious diseases were prevalent, the major concern was survival from the threat of premature death. With increased life expectancy, the quality of life has developed into a prominent component of good health. Health is no longer considered to be merely freedom from life-threatening disease. Because disease has dominated humanity's existence throughout history, the point of view in which health is equated with the absence of disease is readily explainable. This old-fashioned and narrow concept of health is no longer considered adequate or appropriate (World Health Organization, 1984a). Admittedly, if patients with severe pain and disability were asked to describe their concept of health, many would probably emphasize freedom from disease. However, for much of the population in western society health is a condition involving a subjective sense of positive well-being. When such a state does not exist we or those about us begin to wonder if we are ill and want to know what is wrong.

When we are in an optimal state of good health we are capable of doing what we normally do, we are adapted to our environment, and we feel fulfilled. In other words, we have a sense of physical, social, and psychological well-being. By contrast, ill health involves some lack of well-being which includes not functioning at one's usual level. Some degree of adjustment is necessary and expectations need to be modified.

While illness is closely related to the presence of disease, the relationship of disease and illness is variable. The presence of disease does not necessarily mean that someone is ill. Consider, for example, the well controlled patient with epilepsy or hypertension who supports a family, has friends, and is happy. This person is not ill. Equally, the presence of illness does not necessitate the existence of disease. There are many people who are ill in whom no disease has been diagnosed. These are an important group of individuals and they are in need of care and help in the same way as people ill from a recognized disease. Figure 1.1 illustrates this relationship between illness and disease. Health professionals, particularly doctors, are poorly trained to care for health problems for which a diagnosable disease is not the cause. This is a major source of frustration to both patients and physicians.

The subjective sensation of not being well or the prospect of getting ill is the reality which affects the patient. Prior to this, the presence of an undetected disease in the presymptomatic stage presents no current problems to the patient or doctor. Once abnormal physical signs such as swelling or weakness appear or symptoms develop, the patient is usually considered to be unwell. Initially, symptoms without a diagnosis have a similar effect on the patient except that the doctor's response may vary due to the absence of a satisfactory diagnosis. Illness affecting physical, social, and psychological well-being may appear without an identifiable explanation. When a cause is apparent, this may prove to be a physical disease, but disease is not the only cause of illness. Social circumstances such as the loss of a job, moving to a new town, increased responsibility, and many others may lead to illness. Emotional events such as the death of a friend, a birth, marriage, or disruptive personal relationships may also lead to emotional symptoms and illness. The manifestations of illness are wide and varied. They may be physical in nature, such as pain, weakness, nausea. They may be social in nature and affect one's ability to establish, develop, and maintain social contacts. Emotional manifestations range from depression to abnormal elation and include fear, anxiety, agitation, and changes in mood and attitude.

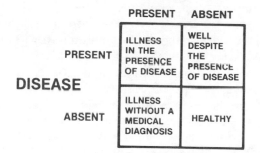

FIGURE 1.1 The relationship of illness and disease.

Disease is better understood than illness, and for this reason medical treatment is dominated by therapies for specific diagnoses. Some of these therapies are effective and others are not. The importance of disease is its ability to disrupt people's lives by making them ill and by the direct effect of disease on survival. As with illness, the type of impact resulting from disease may be physical, social, or psychological. The extent of these potential consequences is particularly relevant to the patient and has been described in detail by the World Health Organization (1980). Disease may lead to impairment through a disturbance or inter- ference with the structure or function of the body and yet not lead to disability. Disability, on the other hand, refers to the loss or reduction of functional ability and activity. Examples of disa- bilities are hearing loss, speech difficulty, inability to enter an elevator, inability to drive a car. When impairment or disability cause a social disadvantage, the patient is said to be handicapped. Handicap is avoided when the patient successfully adapts to his or her impairment or disability. A handicap may be one of immobility which prevents the patient moving from one place to another. However, a wheelchair-bound patient with multiple scle- rosis who can drive a car and transfer independently is impaired and disabled but is not handicapped in terms of mobility. A person who is incapable of providing economically for him- or herself has a self-sufficiency handicap. Other types of handicap include an inability to provide basic physical care for oneself (self-care handicap), a lack of orientation in time or place or person (ori- entation handicap), inability to occupy one's time (occupation handicap), and the inability to make and maintain social relation- ships (social handicap). Disease is a major cause of handicap, although it is not the only cause.

In order to describe the health of a population completely, there are a number of perspectives which should be taken into account. In Figure 1.2 the progression from a subjectively healthy state through the development of symptoms to the consequences of illness in everyday life serves to illustrate three perspectives on health which will be discussed at length in subsequent chapters. Prior to the development of abnormal symptoms a number of factors which predispose to illness may be identifiable. Factors such as smoking, excessive alcohol intake, overeating, and being single or elderly all increase one's risk of illness. The prevalence of such factors, therefore, represents an important dimension to the health of a community. A second dimension is the frequency

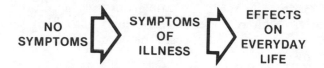

FIGURE 1.2 Three stages of illness (For a detailed description of these stages see White, 1981).

of disease itself. The third dimension is the behavioral manifestation of illness in terms of physical, social, or psychological dysfunction. A common form of physical ill health is reduced agility and immobility. The term social ill health can have a wider meaning than is employed in this book. Social health will be considered in a limited sense and will refer to the nature, extent, and quality of social contacts. Emotional health likewise will be used in a somewhat restricted way and will refer to the individual's subjective feelings and attitudes. In general, this concept of health is one which considers the quality of life as much a part of health as the absence of disease.

Population

The concept of population as it applies to population health has been developed principally by the disciplines of statistics and epidemiology. One of its first demonstrated uses was in the construction of life tables to calculate life expectancy in the 17th century. The application of the concept of population in the health field since then has grown considerably.

Despite improvements in the standard of living and in life expectancy, there remain many inequalities in the distribution of health within society. The identification of health problems within the total population goes only part way to disclosing such inequalities. The health of specific subgroups within society needs to be known so that their health status can be compared with that of the whole society. The term "population" in population health is not restricted to describe the total population, although it has been used principally for this purpose. As the health of subpopulations within society is studied, it becomes easier to focus attention and resources on groups with the most need. This method avoids concealing the serious problems of a minority group within the favorable statistics of the majority.

Populations can be defined in numerous ways. The most common has been the geographically defined population, such as the total population of a province, state, or city. Within a population

defined territorially there are numerous subpopulations such as
the elderly, children under 5 years, men with high serum cholesterol, women with osteoporosis, the poor, the physically disabled,
and so on.

There are several reasons for defining populations so specifically.
The first has already been mentioned, namely, to define precisely
the health needs of a given group. The second is an extension
of this. In order to make valid comparisons in the frequency of
health problems between various groups, it is necessary to know
the population within which the problems occur. The need for
this epidemiological strategy will be described in the next chapter.
Third, consideration of the population to which an individual
belongs can help explain observations. For example, it is observed
that an old man of 86 years has been a smoker all his life. Does
this mean cigarettes do no harm? Think of the population of
which he is a member. Of all the men born in 1900 who have
smoked all their lives the vast majority are dead. Therefore this
old man is an exception and not typical. Finally, the concept of
subgroups helps define therapy more precisely. For example, a
student learns that bacterial sore throats should be treated with
penicillin. However, individuals with bacterial sore throats are not
homogeneous and the bacteria causing pharyngitis are not all the
same. There is a subgroup of individuals who are allergic to
penicillin, although the majority are not. In the case of bacteria,
most are sensitive to penicillin but some are resistant. Therefore
the student should know which patients to treat with penicillin
as well as the distinguishing features of the other groups of patients
who should be treated with an antibiotic other than penicillin.

The definition of health problems in terms of the population
within which they occur allows for increased precision in the
definition of problems; this facilitates comparisons between groups,
helps in the interpretation of observations, and also guides us in
our choice of management. These concepts of health and population provide a method of thinking about health problems.

THE SCIENTIFIC BASIS OF POPULATION HEALTH

Introduction

Employing a scientific method to improve the validity of medical
inference dates back at least 100 years. Late in the 19th century,
when bacteria were responsible for the majority of deaths and

disability, much medical thought focused on identifying the microorganisms responsible for given diseases. In order to facilitate valid conclusions about the etiological relationship between a given microorganism and disease, the German physician Robert Koch (Volk & Wheeler, 1984) defined four criteria, all of which should be met in order to draw this conclusion. Koch postulated that: (1) the microorganism must be regularly isolated from cases of the illness; (2) that it must be grown in pure culture *in vitro*; (3) that when such a pure culture is inoculated into susceptible animal species, the typical disease must result; (4) and that from such experimentally induced disease, the mircoorganism must again be isolated. The application of these criteria prevented overly zealous observers from attributing diseases to particular organisms incorrectly. A similar risk exists with physicians attributing improvements in patients to a particular therapy, and in recent times there has been increased attention to the quality of medical evidence (Hill, 1977, pp. 254–296).

Many decisions in medicine have become accepted practice without being assessed by adequate criteria. One such example was the prescription of bed rest for patients suffering a heart attack (Johnson, 1979). It was accepted by the medical profession in the 1940s and in much of the 1950s that 4 to 6 weeks' bed rest would lead to better healing of the damaged heart than a shorter period of bed rest. This therapeutic decision had not been arrived at in a sufficiently scientific manner. The decision was based on histological knowledge of the healing heart muscle following infarction. From this evidence it was inferred that rest helps the healing of damaged tissue and that rest in bed provides maximal rest for the heart. Mallory, White, and Salcedo-Salgar (1939, p. 670) stated that ". . . our findings support the more or less empirical custom of those who advise for patients with small-to-moderate size myocardial infarcts, without complications, one month of rest in bed . . ., and one month of very carefully graded convalescence, with a third month to consolidate recovery . . . ". This approach to patient management was to change. In 1951, Levine and Lown (1951) published results of a study entitled "The 'Chair' Treatment of Acute Coronary Thrombosis." In this non-controlled experiment, 64 patients with acute myocardial infarction were each put in a chair for increasing portions of the day shortly after admission. The majority of patients were in a Harvard teaching hospital, while the remainder were either at home or in other hospitals. The patients experienced an 11% mortality rate. There was no comparison with a group who did not receive chair treatment. On the basis of this study, and advances in the understanding of pulmonary and cardiac hemodynamics, the authors inferred that chair rest is preferred treatment to strict bed rest for patients with acute coronary thrombosis. Subsequently the amount of bed rest for these patients was reduced progressively. With continued interest in the subject a number of randomized controlled trials have been conducted to test the effect of the duration of bed rest on recovery. No difference was found between study and control groups in these trials (Glasgow Royal Infirmary, 1973; Harpur et al., 1971; Hayes, Morris, and Hampton, 1974; Hutter et al., 1973; McNeer et al., 1978). It has been pointed out, however, that the number of patients in these studies was insufficient to be confident in the findings (Johnson, 1979). Today, patients with uncomplicated heart attacks are mobilized early and strict bed rest is no longer prescribed routinely following the first 24 hours. The relationship between bed rest and recovery in myocardial infarction is just one example in medicine where beliefs and practices have been based on inadequate evidence. No criteria were applied to evaluate the validity of the original practice of prolonged bed rest, and, likewise, the chair treatment was accepted without methodologically sound scrutiny.

There are at least two lessons to be learned from the bed rest story. The first is the need to be aware of the importance of examining the evidence which underlies a given decision. One can surmise that the attitude of the medical profession toward the treatment of myocardial infarction in the 1940s was to turn to the leading medical scientists for leadership, to obtain their opinions, and to accept them without question or without examining the evidence underlying their opinions. While the histological observations of Mallory et al. (1939) were valid, their inference concerning bed rest did not follow. The second lesson is that there is a need for criteria by which to appraise evidence in the way that Koch did for evidence concerning bacterial pathogenesis.

The quality of evidence and the appropriateness of interpretations made from data are of particular importance to the management of health problems in society. Within a population perspective, health data serve three broad purposes, and for each there are particular methodological considerations.

Measuring the Problem

The first task is to define the problem. This involves several steps. The population, or groups to be assessed, needs to be identified precisely. It needs to be decided what aspect of health will be described—deaths, disease frequency, functional health status, or quality of life. Instruments that can measure these characteristics accurately must be selected, and if they are not available, then appropriate data gathering instruments must be developed. The assessment of the prevalence and frequency distribution of health problems is the domain of vital statistics and descriptive epidemiology. These methods help define both the existence of a problem and the sectors of society involved. This is the subject of the next two chapters.

Understanding the Problem

The second task is to understand the problem. Why has it occurred? What factors predispose to it? Ideally, the cause of an illness or disability can be found, but in most instances the best that can be done is to identify risk factors which are associated with an increased frequency of the problem. The task of investigating causation and risk is difficult and is usually a long process. This requires following groups of individuals for periods of time to see who becomes ill. Such prospective studies are a major part of analytic epidemiology. Once a risk factor or a causative agent has been identified this does not mean we know which strategies or interventions will prevent or cure the illness. Chapters 4, 5, and 6 are devoted to this aspect of population health.

Solving the Problem

The third task is identification of effective interventions; this requires the direct evaluation of therapeutic maneuvers and programs by controlled trials. As has been illustrated above, such evidence is not always available; in fact, a large proportion of the interventions used to manage society's health problems have not been tested adequately. Intervention trials are a very precise form of investigation, the design of which has been refined considerably in the last 30 years. Such studies require the specific description of the study population, the problem being treated, the maneuver, the outcomes, and the criteria for success of the trial. Our understanding of solving health problems is the focus of Chapters 7, 8, and 9.

Discussion

The quality of health decisions and policy depends heavily upon the nature and quality of available evidence. It is therefore in the best interest of the population in general that we understand as much as possible about the size and extent of the community's health problems, their causation, and methods to solve them. The evidence in these three areas forms the scientific basis of population health. However, it is important that I do not convey the impression that health policy is primarily a scientific process. The amount of science in public policy and in much medical practice is often small. There are several reasons for this.

POPULATION HEALTH IN PRACTICE

The Inadequacy of Available Data

In addition to having an understanding of the ideal data required, society must cope with the inadequacies of available data. Health professionals and policy makers work routinely with data which are deficient in a variety of ways.

Certain aspects of health are better documented than others. Statistics on deaths, life expectancy, and the diseases causing death are usually well documented and are available on the whole population. Data on the occurrence of disease tend to be measured less frequently, if at all. The United States has tended to be the most progressive in maintaining a record of community morbidity. The quality of life and most of the behavioral aspects of illness are very poorly evaluated, and most often these types of data are only available from surveys of small sectors of society.

The most readily available health data describe the total population according to age, sex, and region. Health data on ethnic, social class, and occupational subgroups are often restricted in availability or do not exist. Our understanding of more specific groups, such as the physically handicapped or individuals with mental illness or arthritis, for example, comes from surveys or clinic registers or agency records.

The cause of disease has been the principal focus of medical research for centuries. To some degree this form of investigation has become more complex and frustrating during this century. The specific bacterial or parasitic causes of so many infectious diseases gave their investigation a finite quality. Chronic disease, on the other hand, appears to be multifactorial in etiology, involving a complex interaction of a variety of risk factors. There are no precise answers to what causes the majority of chronic disorders.

Knowledge of how to prevent and cure illness is also incomplete and quite inadequate. Of course there have been medical successes, as attested by the relative or absolute conquest of diseases such as smallpox, tetanus, polio, diphtheria, phenylketonuria, pernicious anemia, tuberculous meningitis, pneumonia, scurvy, hypertension, and others. This leaves diseases such as arthritis, cancer, heart disease, degenerative neurological disorders, and illnesses such as mental illness, psychological handicaps, and social ill health as outstanding examples of where therapeutic interventions have had little or no beneficial impact.

The Ethics of Health Decisions

The increase in moral consciousness in society and acknowledgment of the moral right of individuals have made ethics a major consideration in health decisions. The ethics of a given decision are a subjective judgement and therefore differ greatly from the methodological factors discussed above (Thomas, 1983, pp. 3–34).

Ethical considerations arise when there is a significantly different value placed on alternative decisions. For example, one decision is considered benevolent yet costly, whereas an alternative decision is judged to be unkind although money-saving. It is a value judgement as to which to choose. A situation where it is necessary to make such choices arises only when resources are limited and the benefits are unavailable to everyone. This is the case in health care, where services are expensive and scarce and the need for care is great. Ethics is concerned with how decisions under these circumstances are made and the process whereby different values involved in a given decision are acknowledged and respected. The decision itself is not of ethical concern.

Ethics has become a major factor in medical decisions for several reasons. The increased sophistication of medicine now offers opportunities for the prolongation of life and for the withdrawal of life supports that used not to exist. Costs are so high that medical services cannot be offered to everyone. Budgeting for the introduction of new programs often results in cutbacks for existing services. The medical benefits of competing technologies involve different values, and the ethical problem becomes one of choosing between two dissimilar services or between two lines of action with incomparable benefits. The predicament is one in which a valued and just cause is denied. How can distributive justice be achieved and be seen to be achieved? The role of ethics is to facilitate decision making that does justice to two worthy points of view of which only one can actually benefit. Therefore, the emphasis is placed on the process of decision making. The following examples illustrate the dilemma.

1. Renal dialysis machines in a particular locality are all occupied except one. Two patients are being considered for the vacant machine; one is a single man, a highly productive research scientist, and the other is a single parent of two young children. Other factors are equal. How should the decision be made? The value of the scientist is to society in general through his research, while the value of the parent is to his two children. Only one can benefit at the expense of the other.

2. An obstetrician delivers an Asian baby who is put up for adoption. There are two families on the doctor's list; how should he choose which one will receive the baby? The first is a Chinese couple with three children; they are bereaving a recent stillbirth. The other couple is white, with no children and no prospect of pregnancy.

3. A 60-year-old woman with severe heart disease has been treated aggressively in a hospital where she is isolated from family and friends. The prognosis is poor. How should the doctor decide when to start treating the patient conservatively in the comfort of her own house and family?

4. Smoking is known to cause more than 90% of all lung cancer. However, the tobacco industry is an important component of the economy. It is decided that only a small antismoking campaign will be funded while the chest surgery facilities in the state are modernized and increased. In this decision, greater value is placed on the treatment of an incurable disease than on its prevention, despite excellent evidence concerning its preventability.

5. Drinking and driving present another value-laden problem. Despite good evidence that drinking causes road deaths and that strict legislation can reduce alcohol-related road fatalities, drinking behavior in many countries is relatively uncurbed. The choice for

government is between the unpopularity of increased regulation and reduced alcohol sales on the one hand, and a high road accident death rate on the other. Many countries prefer the latter.

These are a small sample of a growing number of ethical problems facing the health field. The many other areas not mentioned here include occupational hazard regulation; abortion clinics; the food industry and heart disease; life support systems and the terminally ill; artificial insemination; and many more.

The challenge of medical ethics is to find criteria for moral decision making. These criteria need to be based on the current values and attitudes of society, which define the perceived strengths and weaknesses of each decision. Given the diversity of society, the values placed on any single decision are usually variable. For example, to some people abortion is a moral and humane act whereas to others it is murder. An ethical decision on abortion would be one which acknowledges these two poles of moral judgement and defines a method, acceptable to society, outlining how specific cases would be handled. The ethical aspects of health decisions are of major importance and need to be integrated with the scientific aspects of health care. The way this occurs is largely through the political process.

Health Decisions as a Political Process

Health policy develops from a complex process of influence exerted by a number of sectors of society representing the public, the health professions, the government, patient groups, universities, and various lobby groups. The process is poorly understood; this makes it difficult to monitor and modify.

The greatest influence on health policy has come from the medical profession. The autonomy and dominance of the profession over medical practice has been energetically guarded (Coburn, Torrance, and Kaufert, 1983; Freidson, 1970). Standards of practice and the administration of medical associations have been controlled and evaluated nearly exclusively by doctors. This has led to a growing conflict with governments that have recognized this effective monopoly and have set out to take over some of this control. Consequently, health policy is the result of often tense negotiations between government and the medical profession.

Added to this government–profession axis are a number of other influences. Major health problems, if adequately documented and publicized, often form the focus of influential health lobbies. These forces have varying degrees of success in molding health policy. Examples of problems which have led to important lobbies include occupational hazards in the mining and asbestos industries, air and water pollution, alcohol-related road accidents, exposure to irradiation, inadequacy of health care for specific socioeconomic groups, and many more. These lobbies have also occurred over ethical and human rights issues of which abortion and nuclear arms are noted examples. Lobby groups tend to use public fora and direct contact with government to make their views known. There are also new influences arising from within the professions which are often directed at the professions themselves.

Medical research and academic publications present new views and evidence on health policy. The influence of this type of information is usually slow to occur or may not result in any change at all. The methodological theme of this book is one manifestation of an extensive lobby within the medical profession to place increasing importance on scientific evidence and less on opinion.

SUMMARY

In order to have an unbiased view of health our understanding needs to be both comprehensive and factual. The framework of population health used in this book is designed to reflect both these qualities. Health is considered in a broad sense to include social and psychological well-being as well as physical illness and disease. This holistic view contrasts with the often criticized disease orientation, which is typical of the biomedical concept of health. Health status is highly variable from one group to another, from one age to another, and from ethnic group to ethnic group. Populations of relevance to population health may be big or small and can be defined in terms of many sociodemographic, economic, educational, racial or disease characteristics.

The scientific basis of health policy has been described according to the three major types of health data used in decision making. First, the problem should be described according to the type of health problem and the population affected. Then some understanding of what has caused the problem can form the basis for identifying interventions to be tested as possible solutions to the problem. The evidence presented in the subsequent chapters is arranged according to the three broad categories of problems, causes, and solutions. While ethical and political factors also affect health policy, these factors do not form the principal focus of the text.

Chapter 2

The Problem: A General Perspective on Health

No single measure can describe adequately the health of a community. Only through using a number of indices can a reasonably complete picture of a population's health be constructed. The most easily measured indicator is mortality. This is the end result of disease or injury and does not reflect accurately the antecedent disability which preceded death. The frequency of disease is another commonly employed measure. This provides an added perspective but is limited by a predominatly physical focus. The psychological, social, and occupational aspects of poor health and disability are of great importance to patients but are difficult to measure. For this reason, the behavioral aspects of health tend to be poorly described.

In this chapter a general picture of health at the national level will be presented. This will include both physical and behavioral perspectives. To provide continuity, the data presented are principally but not exclusively North American. Hopefully these data will provide an illustration of the diverse nature of health, the magnitude of the problems, and the trends that are occurring. The gaps in the available information reflect some important realities in society, such as the different values placed on the various aspects of health and the wide range in current methods of measuring health and illness.

The first section deals with methodology and data concerning life expectancy, mortality, and the frequency of disease. The behavioral aspects of health and disability are described in the second section.

The data have been obtained from three sources: vital statistics, which are gathered routinely from the whole population; health record data gathered by health services on patients; and survey data describing selected study populations.

DISEASE

Life Expectancy

Life expectancy has gone through dramatic changes in recent times, and it is easily forgotten how commonly friends and family used to be lost through early death. Consider the history of the Brontë family. Charlotte Brontë was 5 years old when her mother died of cancer. Four years later, her two elder sisters died of tuberculosis not long after they started at boarding school. When Charlotte was 32, she lost her two sisters, Emily and Anne, and her brother, Branwell, all from tuberculosis. In her late thirties she married, but within months she was dead, due either to her pregnancy or tuberculosis. Her father, by contrast, survived to 84. Today, the likelihood of such a history is very small.

Although life expectancy has increased, the human life span has remained constant (Comfort, 1979, pp. 81–86); that is, the proportion of the population reaching old age has increased, but the maximum length of human life is unchanged. Each animal species has its own characteristic life span. This indicates that the ultimate limit to longevity is controlled biologically, through genetic makeup, and is unaffected by environment.

Methodology

The term "life expectancy" is not concerned with this biological programming of the life span. Rather, it describes the likelihood of surviving to a given age at a given time in history. Life expectancy differs from one period to another and from country to country.

Life expectancy is the average (mean) number of years for which a group of individuals of the same age (an age "cohort") are expected to live. Most commonly it refers to life expectancy at birth, but when specified, it can refer to the expected length of life remaining at any age. The years of life expected are calculated from the age-specific death rates of the population which pertain at the time. The importance of life expectancy is not only that it indicates the anticipated duration of life, but it is also a general index of the standard of living.

The Evidence

Life expectancy in North America is slightly higher in Canada than in the United States. In 1980 the expected length of life for males was 71.4 years in Canada and 70.1 years in the United States, for females, it is 78.9 and 77.8 years respectively (World Health Organization, 1984b, pp. 38–39). For both sexes there is a continuing trend for life expectancy to increase. This is greater for females than males, as is the case universally. The largest improvement has occurred in life expectancy at birth, with successively smaller improvements at all subsequent ages. Here too the gains for females surpass those for males. For example, at 65 years of age life expectancy for U.S. males increased by 2.9 years between 1900–1902 and 1982, while the increase for females was 6.0 years (National Center for Health Statistics, 1983a, p. 99).

The probability of living can be expressed either in terms of survival or mortality. Life expectancy takes a positive perspective, whereas mortality rates describe the likelihood of dying. As people are mortal, there is not a question of whether or not a person will die; it is only a question of when death will occur.

Mortality

The measurement of mortality is probably the most direct and fundamental method to assess the health status of a population. A mortality rate's limitation is the inability to reflect quality of life and disability. Concern with preventing death has had a long history and in the past has been equated justifiably with health. For example, in the pre-antibiotic era a child who survived a life-threatening episode of measles or pneumonia had a probability of surviving to old age comparable to someone who had not been similarly afflicted. Energetic efforts to prevent death from these conditions had the potential of being highly rewarding. In current times, when the majority of disease affects the elderly, similar therapeutic vigor to avoid death can be carried to a point when dehumanizing measures have very little influence on prolonging useful life. This creates a moral conflict in which decisions to sustain life in biological terms compete with concern for the quality of life. For modern medicine this remains an unresolved ethical dilemma.

Methodology

Despite the fact that death is a readily identifiable outcome, the measurement of the occurrence of death deserves specific consideration. The methodological aspects of mortality will be considered by means of a simple problem.

The problem: In a retirement village by the sea it is observed that the mortality rate exceeds that in a new suburban subdivision on the outskirts of a nearby city. Does this mean that the state of health is lower in the retirement village?

The key concept to understanding mortality is that death rates and the age composition of a population should be considered together. Gross errors can arise from considering mortality in isolation. In addition to the ethical problem mentioned above, there are methodological reasons for grouping these two concepts. Let us examine the reasons for this.

The older a person is, the more likely he or she is to die. A boy in 1976 between the age of 1 and 14 years had a 1 in 2,000 chance of dying. By contrast, the likelihood of death in an elderly man aged between 70 and 79 in the same year was 100 times greater. The respective death rates for the two age groups were 0.48 per 1,000 per year and 48 per 1,000 per year (Wilkins, 1980a, p. 30).

These are age-specific death rates. This type of rate is the proportion of all deaths of individuals of a given age during a given year to the total mid-year population of individuals of the same age.

Consider the age structure of the retirement village and the new subdivision. In the village the age ranges upward from 50 years, whereas the subdivision is occupied by young families, with few elderly people. Given that age-specific death rates for old people far exceed those for the young, the difference in age composition of the two communities could explain the difference in death rate. The age structure of a population is usually the principal determinant of the overall mortality rate (crude death rate).

The crude death rate (CDR) is the proportion of all deaths to the total population in one year. Usually this proportion is multiplied by 1000 so the CDR expresses the number of deaths per 1000 population per year.

The effect of age on death is of little practical importance because this relationship cannot be modified. By contrast, there are other factors which are potentially alterable. For this reason it is important to detect differences in death rates due to factors other than the biological effect of age. If two groups of individuals of the same age have different death rates, one can assume that this difference is due to something other than age. A true difference in age-specific death rates is indicative of a difference in health status.

In comparing the health status of the retirement village and the new subdivision, the question is whether the difference in crude death rates is explained completely by age composition, or whether age-specific death rates are also different.

The crude death rate of a population depends upon two factors: first, the age composition, and second, the age-specific death rates for each age group of the population. In order that comparisons of mortality between populations can be used to indicate differences in health status, and not simply differences in age composition, it is important to employ a measure of death which controls either one of these two factors. There are several ways in which this can be done. The most precise method is to compare directly the age-specific death rates. The drawback of this is that it can be cumbersome. Second, the statistical technique of standardization (adjustment) can be used. There are two types of standardization. Direct standardization controls age composition by applying the age-specific rates of the populations being compared to a single standard population. The resulting death rate is called an age-standardized or age-adjusted death rate. Because a standard population and not the actual population has been used in the calculation, the standardized rate is artificial, and can be employed only for comparing the two populations from which the age-specific death rates were obtained. The other method of standardization is the indirect method, which controls both age-specific death rates and age composition and generates a ratio of two death rates called the standardized mortality ratio (SMR). The numerator is the observed or actual death rate in a given population, and the denominator is the hypothetical death rate in that population, had the age-specific death rates of a comparison population been in effect. When there is no difference between the two populations, that is, the observed and expected death rates are equal, the SMR = 1, or 100%. When the observed population has a higher mortality (is less healthy), the SMR > 1 or > 100%. Finally, an SMR <

1 or < 100% indicates that the observed population is more healthy. A third but less practical means for reducing inaccuracies in comparing death rates is to compare the crude rates only of populations with similar age compositions.

Measures of mortality provide a general overview of the health of a country or a population. Crude death rates are used for this purpose when comparing many countries with one another. Such a general overview is adequately served by the CDR despite its recognized inaccuracies. More informative, however, are international comparisons of selected age-specific death rates, the most useful of which is the infant mortality rate.

The infant mortality rate is the proportion of all deaths of liveborn babies between birth and one year of age over all live births in a given year multiplied by 1000.

Age-specific death rates are just one type of specific death rate. For comparisons within countries and between particular groups, the specific death rate can be most useful. Death rates used in this way include rates specific to variables such as sex, marital status, social class, race, occupation, smoking habits, immunization status, and so on.

Death rates have important limitations. A death rate is a direct measure of the event of death, but is only a weak and indirect measure of the morbidity leading to death. Second, a death rate is only an average or mean estimate and therefore variations in the risk of dying within a population can be concealed. This is most likely with crude death rates but can occur also with age-adjusted and age-specific rates. With an age-specific rate, for example, variations in death rate with sex and social class cannot be identified. An age–sex–social class-specific death rate would be needed to identify such variation.

The Evidence

Accompanying the increase in life expectancy, there has been a steady decline in mortality which has been documented from the first routinely available mortality statistics in 1900 in the United States (10 states and the District of Columbia) and in 1921 in Canada. A similar trend has occurred in the other developed countries (Leacy, 1983, pp. 7–9). By 1983, the crude mortality rate was down to 8.6 per 1,000 per year in the United States (World

Health Organization, 1984b, p. 28) and 7.0 per 1,000 per year in
Canada (Statistics Canada, 1985, p. 2).

The J-shaped age distribution of mortality displayed in Figure
2.1 illustrates two peaks, one at birth and the other starting in
late middle age. Following a small peak in deaths during the first
days and weeks of life, the death rate falls to a very low plateau
that is maintained through the first five decades. After age 50
deaths start to climb, and by age 60 an exponential increase in
the death rate begins. This peak far exceeds that following birth.
A century ago this curve was relatively flat. Deaths used to occur
at a more or less steady rate throughout life, so the deaths of
those who now survive to old age were distributed across all age
groups.

Causes of Death

Understanding the causes of death in industrialized society is
primarily an exercise in understanding chronic disease and accidents. Chronic diseases are generally degenerative in nature, many
of which result from exaggeration of the biological processes of
aging. This applies to diseases such as cancer, cardiovascular disease,
cerebrovascular disease, some respiratory diseases, and osteoar-
thritis.

The leading causes of death in the United States (National
Center for Health Statistics, 1984a, p. 6) (Table 2.1), as in most
developed countries, are ischemic heart disease, cancer, stroke,
and accidents. These are mainly diseases of the elderly, with some
notable exceptions. Heart disease and female cancers start to appear

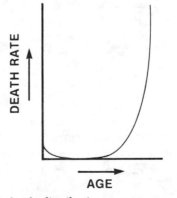

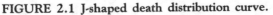

FIGURE 2.1 J-shaped death distribution curve.

as important causes of death around the age of 40. Stroke, on the other hand, peaks after age 65. Accidental deaths and suicide affect all ages but are of greater frequency in the young.

Within this general pattern there are big differences in mortality between males and females. Early death is mainly a male problem. In the case of death from accidents, in 1979 the age-adjusted death rates in the United States for males and females, respectively, were 66.2 and 22.4 per 100,000 per year (National Center for Health Statistics, 1984a, p. 8), and in Canada 100.1 and 39.9 per 100,000 per year (Statistics Canada, 1982a, pp. 20, 22), respectively. Heart disease also affects more males than females. In the case of neoplasm, the death rate from lung cancer in the United States in 1979 was 59.3 per 100,000 per year for males and 17.3 per 100,000 per year for females (National Center for Health Statistics, 1984a, p. 8). The Canadian figures are very similar (Statistics Canada, 1982a, pp. 20, 22). There are indications that these sex differences in lung cancer are changing with alterations in the smoking habits of males and females.

While the overall death rate has been declining steadily, the deaths from some causes have remained static for many years,

TABLE 2.1: Major Causes of Death, United States, 1979 (Crude Death Rates per 100,000)

Causes of Death in Rank Order	Rate	% of Total Deaths
1. Diseases of heart	333.1	38.3
2. Malignant neoplasms	183.3	21.1
3. Cerebrovascular diseases	77.0	8.9
4. Accidents & adverse effects	47.8	5.5
5. Chronic obstructive pulmonary diseases & allied conditions	22.7	2.6
6. Pneumonia & influenza	20.5	2.4
7. Diabetes mellitus	15.1	1.7
8. Chronic liver disease & cirrhosis	13.5	1.6
9. Atherosclerosis	13.1	1.5
10. Suicide	12.4	1.4
11. Certain conditions originating in the perinatal period	10.7	1.2
12. Homicide & legal intervention	10.2	1.2
13. Nephritis, nephrotic syndrome, & nephrosis	7.1	0.8
14. Congenital anomalies	6.1	0.7
15. Septicaemia	3.6	0.4
All other causes	93.3	10.7

Source: National Center for Health Statistics, 1984a, p. 6.

others have increased, and some of the major causes of death are now showing signs of decline. First consider heart disease, one of the major epidemics of the 20th century. The death rate from ischemic heart disease climbed progressively from the early 1900s up to approximately 1960. It has been declining since then (Stallones, 1980). Deaths from stroke have not had the same epidemic rise as heart disease, but have shown a recent fall (Soltero et al, 1978). Motor vehicle deaths are now showing signs of a decline (National Center for Health Statistics, 1983a, p. 256).

The trend in cancer mortality is more complex because of important differences in the secular trend of respiratory and non-respiratory cancers and because of differences between men and women. In the United States these trends have been analyzed in detail by Doll and Peto (1981). The one form of cancer that is increasing markedly is lung cancer. All others are either approximately constant or declining. Lung cancer deaths are increasing among females of all ages and in males over 49 years. Cancers which are more or less constant are nonrespiratory cancers in men. Female mortality from nonrespiratory cancer is falling steadily, and since the mid-1970's lung cancer mortality rates for males under 49 years have also been falling (Doll and Peto, 1981, pp. 1207–1211, 1295). (As will be discussed subsequently, the mortality rates from cancer differ in some instances from incidence rates.)

There has been a steady decline throughout this century for all causes of death among neonates (aged from birth to 28 days) and infants (aged from birth to 1 year). The infant mortality rate in the United States fell from 95.7 in 1915–1919 to 13.1 in 1979 (National Center for Health Statistics, 1984a, Sec. 2, p. 1) and in Canada from 104.3 in 1922 to 9.6 in 1981 (Wilkins, 1980a, p. 30; Statistics Canada,1981a, Table 19). The greatest decline occurred in the postneonatal period (from 28 days to 1 year of age) due to the reduction in infectious disease deaths. Early this century, 55% of all infant deaths occurred after the first 28 days of life, whereas by 1979 only 32% of infant deaths were postneonatal (National Center for Health Statistics, 1984a, Sec. 2, p. 1). Most neonatal deaths now occur in the first week of life (early neonatal period) (Statistics Canada, 1981a, Table 1). The major cause of both stillbirths and early neonatal deaths is prematurity. It is for this reason that the perinatal death rate is being used increasingly in preference to rates which do not include stillbirths.

The perinatal death rate is the proportion of all fetal deaths aged 28 weeks and over plus all neonatal deaths in the first week of life over all live births plus stillbirths expressed per 1000 per year.

The impact of a disease upon society is only partially reflected in the mortality rate. The other factor to consider, as mentioned above, is the age at which the deaths occur. The age distribution of given causes of death will affect the years of life lost due to disease. Although the death rate from accidents is fourth in order of magnitude (being less than heart disease, cancer, and stroke), in Canada motor vehicle accidents are the leading cause of years of life lost (Lalonde, 1974, p. 15).

Disease Frequency

Many health problems and diseases do not cause death and consequently are not reflected in mortality statistics. Many of these nonlethal diseases account for much of the suffering and inconvenience experienced by patients and for this reason need to be estimated.

To this point we have dealt with the probability of survival and the frequency of death. To a major degree these parameters are the resultant effects of disease. The focus will now change from these major outcomes to the disease itself. However, the measurement of disease status in the community is relatively crude and imprecise.

While death certificates permit mortality statistics to be compiled routinely on the total population, there is not a comparable method for the collection of morbidity statistics. The principal method for obtaining population-based morbidity data is a national health survey based on a sample of the population. Such surveys are carried out routinely in the United States and Britain. In Canada there was the Canadian Sickness Survey in 1951, which was followed by the Canada Health Survey during 1978 and 1979 (Statistics Canada, 1981b). Other sources of community morbidity data are registers for particular diseases such as cancer, diabetes, multiple sclerosis, Huntington's chorea, and muscular dystrophy, among others. Indirect measures of disease frequency are the utilization statistics of health services.

In the United States National Health Interview Survey (NHIS) a probability sample of households in the civilian noninstitutionalized population is interviewed each week of the year. In 1981 the sample was composed of approximately 41,000 households containing about 107,000 persons. Approximately 97% responded to the interview (National Center for Health Statistics, 1982, p. 7).

Acute conditions are one aspect of morbidity investigated by the NHIS. Acute conditions are defined as those illnesses and injuries that last less than 3 months and that involve medical attention or 1 day or more of restricted activity. The incidence of acute conditions in 1981 was 212 per 100 persons per year. Respiratory conditions were the most frequent with a rate of 112 per 100 per year, followed in order by injuries (33 per 100 per year), infective and parasitic conditions (24 per 100 per year), and digestive system conditions (10 per 100 per year). All other acute conditions combined had an incidence rate of 34 per 100 per year (National Center for Health Statistics, 1982, p. 2).

The prevalence of mainly chronic conditions, as assessed by the Canadian Health Survey, found rheumatism and joint disease to be the most prevalent disorders, affecting approximately 20% of the Canadian population. Only 4% of those interviewed reported having heart disease (Statistics Canada, 1981b, p. 116). These data demonstrate the marked difference in the pattern of disease causing morbidity and the causes of death, as displayed in Table 2.1.

Turning to disease registry data, let us examine two aspects of the occurrence of cancer. The incidence rates for male and female cancers in Canada are shown in Table 2.2; U. S. rates are similar. Skin cancer is by far the most common cancer; except for melanoma it is rarely a cause of death. Apart from skin cancer the principal malignancy in males is lung cancer. While it has a far lower frequency in females the relative and absolute importance of lung cancer in women is rising. Breast cancer is the most common cancer in women.

In their detailed analysis of the causes of cancer, Doll and Peto (1981) addressed a problem concerning differences between incidence and mortality rates in the U.S. population under 65. Both male and female incidence rates for all cancers, except lung and skin cancer, are increasing, while the mortality rates are declining. The importance of this observation is that if it is valid it could indicate that cancers are becoming less malignant or the cure rate of treatment is improving. They analyzed the data for bowel cancer, breast cancer, and prostate cancer, and concluded that the increased incidence rates do not reflect a true increase in the occurrence

TABLE 2.2: Age-Standardized Incidence Rates (rounded) per 100,000 of the Most Common New Primary Sites of Cancer by Diagnosis and Sex, Canada (minus Ontario), 1979

Male		Female	
Site	Rate	Site	Rate
Skin	70	Breast	73
Lung, bronchus trachea	60	Skin	55
Prostate	46	Colon, rectum	39
Colon, rectum	39	Uterus	18
Bladder	20	Lung, bronchus trachea	15
Mouth, lip	16	Lymphatic hemopoietic	13
Stomach	15	Cervix	12
Lymphatic, hem-opoietic	14	Ovary	12
Pancreas	8	Stomach	8
Leukemia	7	Pancreas	6
All malignant neoplasms	349 per 100,000 per year		303 per 100,000 per year

Source: Statistics Canada 1983a, pp. 26–47.

of these cancers. How could such an artefact in the national U.S. cancer statistics occur? The explanation follows.

In the natural history of many cancers there is a long period during which the cancer is present but is not diagnosed. Diagnosis of cancer usually occurs after the patient notices a lump or abnormal symptoms. At any point in time, therefore, there are people with cancer in the community who are as yet unaware of their cancer. However, these undiagnosed cases could be identified if screened or submitted to a number of medical tests and examinations. What is thought to be happening is that this pool of undiagnosed cancer patients is being diagnosed earlier than usual. The proposed reason for this is that patients and health professions are more aggressive than previously in their efforts to detect cancer. Thus, the rate of diagnosis has increased and this is reflected in higher incidence rates. This also boosts the prevalence of cancer (Doll and Peto, 1981, pp. 1274–1278); however, the true occurrence rate of cancer is unchanged. This phenomenon is referred to as the lead-time obtained by screening, or zero-time shift (Sackett, 1980).

Commonly used indicators of the occurrence of disease are health service utilization statistics, particularly those of hospital usage. In the United States in 1982, 38.6 million inpatients were registered in non-federal short-stay hospitals. The duration of stay for the first-listed diagnostic categories provides a useful index of the burden on hospital care generated by given diseases. Table 2.3 displays the discharge rates and duration of stay for the most common diseases. For all listed diagnoses, diseases of the circulatory system ranked first, followed by diseases of the digestive system, supplementary disease classifications, diseases of the genitourinary system, diseases of the respiratory system, and injury and poisoning. These six groups accounted for 60% of all listed diagnoses for 1982 (National Center for Health Statistics, 1984b, p. 7). While arthritis and musculoskeletal problems constitute the most common disease in the community, these problems are not a leading cause of hospital admission.

DISABILITY

In this section the biomedical focus on death rates and disease frequency is replaced by a more general and behavioral perspective on health status. This perspective is concerned with health in terms of a spectrum which ranges from healthfulness to disability. Unfortunately, the criteria for disability are far fewer and are less developed than for biomedical problems. Disability is not simply the inverse of disease; for this reason it needs to be measured directly. This is illustrated by the fact that not all patients with a disease are disabled and among the disabled there are those individuals for whom no biomedical diagnosis can be made.

There is no single indicator which satisfactorily describes the degree of healthfulness or disability of a society. A variety of measures need to be employed, each providing a description of disability from a different perspective. Such measures include data on: (1) institutionalization, (2) activity restriction, (3) emotional health, (4) social health, (5) the demographic structure of society and (6) morbidity as seen in primary care practice. Data from each of these sources will be considered.

TABLE 2.3: Hospital Discharge Rates and Days of Care for Short-Stay Hospitals by Selected First-Listed Diagnostic Categories, United States, 1982

Diagnostic Category	Discharge Rate Per 1000 Pop.	Days of Care, Percentage of Total Days of Care From All Conditions*
Females with deliveries	17.2	5.2
Heart disease	15.1	11.4
Malignant neoplasms	8.6	8.1
Fractures, all sites	4.9	4.2
Cerebrovascular diseases	3.6	3.7
Pneumonia, all forms	3.6	2.4
Diabetes mellitus	2.9	2.3
Noninfectious enteritis & colitis	2.7	1.2
Benign neoplasms, carcinoma in situ, and neoplasms of uncertain behavior	2.7	1.4
Psychoses	2.5	3.3
Arthropathies & related disorders	2.5	1.8

* Not all conditions are shown in table.
Source: National Center for Health Statistics, 1984b, p. 6.

Institutionalization

Institutionalization commonly involves the separation of people from their usual environment. For some individuals this brings an improvement in their standard of living. However, for most of us life in our own home is preferable to life in a long-term institution. More than three quarters of people admitted to nursing homes in the United States require admission because of poor physical health. Other reasons for admission are psychological, social, and economic. The majority of Americans in long-term institutions are in nursing homes. In 1977, 1.126 million Americans aged 65 years and over were in this type of institution (National Center for Health Statistics, 1981, pp. 6, 8) and 225,805 individuals (in 1978) of all ages were in specialty hospitals (National Center for Health Statistics, 1984c, p. 23). In 1980 about 10% of the population 75 years of age and over were in nursing homes. There is a fourfold variation in this figure between states. Those states with the coldest climate and the smallest black population have the largest census in nursing homes. This may reflect a greater need for institutional care among the elderly in cold climates, as well as the lower admission rates among blacks to long-term institutions (National Center for Health Statistics, 1984d, p. 30).

Activity Restriction

Data on activity restriction come mainly from population survey data. In the National Health Survey disability days are estimated from interviewees' responses to questions concerning the 2-week period prior to the week of the interview. A day of restricted activity is defined as a day on which a person restricted his/her normal activities for the entire day as a result of illness or injury. This day of restricted activity is a bed disability day if the person stayed in bed for more than half of the daylight hours. A work-loss day is a day on which a person did not work at his/her job at least half of their normal workday because of illness of injury. A school-loss day is a normal school day on which a child did not attend school because of illness or injury (National Center for Health Statistics, 1983b, p. 4).

In 1980 the average annual rate of restricted activity in the U.S. civilian noninstitutionalized population was 19.1 days per person. Of these days, an estimated 7.0 days were spent in bed per person per year. These figures are averages; therefore, note that 52.1% of the population had no bed disability days, and 2.7% of the population experienced 31 or more bed days in the year prior to interview (National Center for Health Statistics, 1983b, p. 4). Among Canadians the rate of disability days is slightly less than in the U.S. (Statistics Canada, 1981b, p. 122).

The highest rates of restricted activity, 39.2 days per person per year, and bed disability, 13.8 days per person per year, were among the elderly (65 years of age and over) (National Center for Health Statistics, 1983b, p. 45). Those aged between 5 and 24 years had the lowest rates. Females experienced more activity restriction than men, and blacks more than whites (National Center for Health Statistics, 1983b, pp. 4–5). A similar relationship of age and sex with disability has been observed in Canada (Wilkins and Adams, 1982, pp. 11–12). Currently employed individuals aged 17 to 64 lost 5.0 days from work per person per year. The highest rates were reported among males aged 55 to 64. School-age children, 6 to 16 years old, were absent from school an average of 5.3 days per person per year (National Center for Health Statistics, 1983b, p. 6).

Activity restriction is associated with both family income and self-reported health status. Individuals in families with an annual income below $7,000 have, on average, twice the frequency of activity restricted days as those with an income of $25,000 or more. There is approximately a fivefold excess of activity restricted days among individuals who describe their health as fair or poor compared with those describing their health as excellent or good (National Center for Health Statistics, 1983b, p. 5).

Disability is becoming an increasingly important health problem. The frequency of activity restriction (National Center for Health Statistics, 1983b, p. 4) and long-term institutionalization (National Center for Health Statistics, 1981, p. 4) both increase exponentially with age. This has obvious implications for an aging population. Despite some declines in death rates from heart disease and stroke, there was a 25% increase in long-term disability in the noninstitutionalized American population during the decade 1966–1976 (Colez and Blanchet, 1981). Although life expectancy is increasing, the benefit of the added years of life is potentially offset by the increase in disability with advancing age.

Wilkins and Adams (1982) have addressed the incompleteness of considering life expectancy and disability separately. They have developed an index of health expectancy based on life expectancy, activity restriction, and institutionalization. A weighting is assigned according to the relative value placed on each of the three components.

Emotional Health

In order to assess emotional health many measures have been devised but no clearly superior one has yet been acclaimed.

The Canadian Health Survey (Statistics Canada, 1981b) adopted a basic approach in which emotional well-being was evaluated in terms of the presence of positive affect or good feelings and symptoms of anxiety and depression. It was found that 46% of Canadians 15 years of age and older have positive feelings about their lives. Forty-one percent were neutral or had a mixture of positive and negative feelings, while only 4% had predominantly negative feelings. The same pattern exists for symptoms, only 4% revealing frequent symptoms of anxiety and depression. Although there is a little variation with age and sex some patterns are apparent. Generally, teenagers and the old have slightly lower emotional health than the rest of the population. Females in general have only slightly more negative feelings and symptoms of distress than men. The exceptions to this are in the two age groups, 15 to 19 and 45 to 64, in which the emotional health of women is not as good as that of males (Statistics Canada, 1981b, pp. 129–132).

Nagi (1976) measured emotional performance in the general U.S. population aged 18 years and over. He defines emotional performance as a person's effectiveness in psychological coping with life stress, which can be manifested through levels of anxiety, restlessness, and a variety of symptoms. He found the prevalence of limitations in emotional performance to be 34% for none or minimal limitation, 40% for some, 19% for substantial, and 7% for severe limitations. In contrast to the Canadian rate there was a consistent increase in severe limitations with increasing age, and a more pronounced sex difference in which females consistently had more emotional performance limitations than males. In examining the relationship between emotional performance and general health status it was found that individuals with good physical health had nearly twice the likelihood of having good emotional performance as individuals with poor physical health (Nagi, 1976).

In a study of depression a national sample found the prevalence of depressive symptoms in the United States to be 11% for males and 21% for females, adjusted for race (Eaton and Kessler, 1981). This corresponds quite well with a number of other studies (five in the United States and one in the U.K.) in which the prevalence of these symptoms ranged from 13 to 20% (Boyd and Weissman, 1982).

The consistently higher rates of emotional problems in these studies, compared with Canada, could mean several things. It is possible that there is a true difference and that Canadians are emotionally more healthy than Americans, but other probable explanations should also be considered. One possibility is that the instruments used were not similar so that in these studies different patient attributes were measured. It is also possible that the measurements are biased such that the Canadian data have underestimated the problem, or that other studies have inflated the truth. Finally, the different rates may have arisen from differences in the methods of analysis. The most probable explanation is that some combination of these interpretations applies.

Social Health

As defined earlier, social health is considered the quality and quantity of an individual's relationships with other people. An individual who is dissatisfied with his or her contact with friends and family, and who is rarely involved with others, would be thought of as being in a relatively poor state of social health compared to someone with frequent satisfactory relationships. The measures of social health to be discussed will therefore reflect some aspects of either the frequency or quality of social contacts. Data on these parameters for this purpose are difficult to find and consequently only illustrative examples are described. A comprehensive definition of the social health of society is not available.

In a study of 37,678 Sydney adults, Reynolds, Rizzo, and Gallagher (1981) measured degree of satisfaction with a variety of social relationships. They found 1 in 4 adults were not satisfied with their job, and that 15% of males and 19% of females rated their marriage as fair or not good. Sexual problems were reported in approximately 17% of cases.

In the case of the quantitative aspects of social relationships, Nagi (1976) provides some insight into both involvement in work activities and the need for supportive relationships. He found 10.7% of Americans 18 to 65 years of age to be either limited in work activities or completely disabled and unable to work. These rates were higher in blacks, the widowed, and in separated or divorced individuals. Work disability was closely related to the individual's reported health status. Of individuals reporting fair or poor health, 36% were disabled or limited in work roles and activities compared to 5% of individuals reporting themselves to be in good health (Nagi, 1976).

One indicator of the need for social relationships can be inferred from the Independent Living Index. Based on the need for assistance in activities of daily living Nagi (1976) reported that 5% of the American population is not independent. This is a measure of the need for social relationships for purposes of physical mobility, which is one of several functions fulfilled by social contact.

A study directly measuring social ties and relationships was conducted on the Alameda County population by Berkman and Syme (1979). This was a 9-year prospective study of social networks, host resistance, and mortality among a random sample of 6,928 adults. The sources of social contact measured were marriage, friends and relatives, church membership, and informal and formal group associations. A Social Network Index was employed. The index was based on both the number of social ties and their relative importance; for example, the intimate contact of marriage was given more weight than church membership. The scale ranged from I; the fewest social connections, to IV; the most connections. Forty percent of the population fell into the two lowest categories on the scale. Women tended to be more socially isolated than men (Berkman and Syme, 1979).

The importance of social ties beyond their intrinsic value is borne out by the association with mortality. The death rate in males with the fewest social connections was more than double that in men with the most connections. For females the death rate was nearly three times greater for women with the fewest connections compared with women with the most connections (see Table 2.4). In an effort to explain this association the authors systematically examined various explanations. They concluded that the data are consistent with social networks being casually associated with mortality (Berkman and Syme, 1979).

The Demographic Dimension to Health

Population changes have played a central role in history; the relationship of the recent growth in population to health is one example. The pattern of morbidity seen in western society is closely related to the increasing proportion of elderly people and to the predominance of chronic disease.

In Massachusetts in 1850, life expectancy was only 38.3 years (U.S. Bureau of the Census, 1975, p. 56), so there were very few elderly individuals in the population. With life expectancy having nearly doubled in the ensuing 135 years, the population has become

TABLE 2.4: Age-Adjusted Mortality Rates From all Causes per 100, Ages 30-69, and Social Network Index, Alameda County, 1965–1974

Social Network Index		Males	Females
I	Fewer connections	15.6	12.1
II		12.2	7.2
III		8.6	4.9
IV	Most connections	6.4	4.3
	TOTAL	9.5	6.4

Source: Berkman and Syme, 1979, p. 192.

comparatively old. Demographic projections are that the present aging trend will continue.

The major reason for this demographic change has been the decline in premature mortality. Whereas infant mortality in the United States was 100 per 1,000 live births in 1915, it had fallen dramatically to 20 per 1,000 by 1970. Deaths from infectious diseases, including tuberculosis, respiratory infections, gastrointestinal infections, and communicable diseases, have declined markedly during this century. The death rate from tuberculosis fell from 194.4 to 2.6 deaths per 100,000 between 1900 and 1970 (U.S. Bureau of the Census, 1975, pp. 57–58). No longer does the majority of the population have its normal life span interrupted prematurely. The average North American now lives into the 70s.

When infectious disease was the principal cause of morbidity and mortality, there was a relatively uniform death rate for all age groups. This resulted in the age structure of the population being pyramidal in shape. The base of the pyramid represents the young, with older age groups represented at progressively higher levels ascending to the few remaining elderly at the apex. The age composition of the population can be illustrated graphically by a survival curve, as in Figure 2.2. The highest point on the curve, at the top left corner, represents 100% of the population alive at birth. The curve immediately declines steeply due to high neonatal and infant mortality. Thereafter the slope is gradual and progressive until old age when all have died. The shape of the curve tended towards a linear slope at the time that infectious disease predominated.

In recent times the shape of the curve has been changing. Early death has declined so the slope is now more gradual. This relative plateau persists until around 60 years of age, at which time it becomes increasingly steep. Finally the curve plateaus out again due to the normal bell-shaped distribution of death among individuals who survive to old age. This change in the shape, as shown in Figure 2.2, is referred to as rectangularization of the survival curve (Fries and Crapo, 1981).

This rectangularization is due to the increased proportion of the population surviving to old age. It is important to note that there has not been any change in the life span. With reference to this latter point, it is as though there is a biological wall somewhere about 85 to 100 years of age beyond which men and women cannot survive. The reports of isolated primitive communities with elders living to 140 years of age have been found

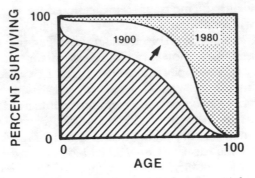

FIGURE 2.2 Linear and rectangular survival curves (Adapted from Fries and Crapo, 1981, p. 73).

to be an artefact resulting from progressively overestimating the age of the elderly (Mazess & Forman, 1979).

The start of the steep decline in the curve around age 60 is due to chronic disease, without which this rapid fall would start further to the right. Despite the longevity of most people, the steady loss of life throughout all ages due to accidents is reflected by the gradual slope in the middle of the curve. This contribution to the curve has undergone little change this century.

A superficial glance at the improvement in survival could leave the impression that everything is much better than previously. Why then is there such concern about geriatrics and health care for the elderly? The answer is twofold. An aging population alone does not imply ill health; however, longevity combined with chronic disease does. So long as chronic disease is prevalent among the middle-aged, the aging population brings the potential of an epidemic of disability and infirmity. It is therefore relevant for the health of aging populations that the onset of chronic disease be postponed if not prevented, and that efforts be made to minimize disability when chronic disease does occur.

Morbidity in Primary Care Practice

The last perspective on morbidity to be described is that seen in primary medical practice. It would seem logical to assume that the profile of presenting complaints in primary care would correspond closely to the morbidity profile of the community. It has been shown, however, that a large proportion of episodes of ill health (two thirds) do not present to the medical care system (White, Williams, & Greenberg, 1961). By the time patients arrive at their physician's office, a selection process has already been in effect. The problems seen in primary care are the ones which patients are asking to have treated and are the only problems to which the medical care system has direct access. The pattern of morbidity seen in general practice is biased by the patient's decision of whether or not to consult a doctor. However, the problems which present in primary care reflect community health more closely than the utilization statistics of secondary and tertiary services to which are referred only a selected subgroup of primary care patients. Statistics on morbidity in general practice have been collected in a number of countries, among which those in Britain and the U.S. are particularly comprehensive. There is a general similarity in the nature and distribution of health problems seen in countries such as Australia, Britain, Canada, and the United States. The reasons for visiting general and family physicians as found in the U.S. National Ambulatory Medical Care Survey (National Center for Health Statistics, 1983c, p. 11) illustrate this general pattern (Table 2.5). The pattern differs in some important ways from data presented earlier, being in some respects a combination of the frequency of disease in the community and the community's perception of its ill health.

Physical examinations, respiratory symptoms, blood pressure measurement, and prenatal assessments are among the leading reasons for consulting primary care physicians. Many consultations are for prophylactic and preventive reasons and many symptoms presented by patients do not reflect recognized diseases. The diagnoses that are made in general practice exclude those visits at which a medical diagnosis is not made. Whereas heart disease, cancer, strokes, and accidents are the leading causes of death, these diseases have a lower frequency among the diagnoses made in primary care than would be inferred from mortality statistics alone (Table 2.6). Disease of the respiratory system is the most common diagnosis category in general practice, followed by diseases of the circulatory system, injury, poisoning, and musculoskeletal disease. The finding that cancers comprise only 1.2% of office visits to general and family physicians (National Center for Health Statistics, 1983c, p. 28) is noteworthy.

The frequency of emotional difficulties and symptoms of mental disability may not be fully evident from these data. Care needs to be taken in interpreting data on the frequency of mental health as a number of factors tend to conceal emotional problems. The stigma of mental illness deters patients from presenting emotional

TABLE 2.5: Percent Distribution of the 20 Most Frequent Principal Reasons
for Office Visits to General and Family Practitioners, United States,
January 1980 to December 1981

Principal Reasons for Visit	%
All visits	100
General medical examination	5.4
Symptoms referable to throat	4.4
Blood pressure test	3.3
Cough	3.0
Head cold, upper respiratory infection (coryza)	2.8
Prenatal examination, routine	2.5
Back symptoms	2.4
Chest pain & related symptoms (not referrable to body system)	2.0
Progress visit, not otherwise specified	1.9
Headache, pain in head	1.9
Hypertension	1.8
Abdominal pain, cramps, spasms	1.7
Skin rash	1.7
Earache, or ear infection	1.6
Vertigo, dizziness	1.5
Fever	1.4
Weight gain	1.2
Well-baby examination	1.1
Lower back symptoms	1.1
Leg symptoms	1.1

Source: National Center for Health Statistics, 1983c, p. 11.

symptoms and enhances the likelihood of a patient complaining
of a physical symptom before admitting to a behavioral problem.
This is facilitated by the frequent association between physical
and emotional symptoms. From the doctor's perspective the body
is easier to understand and treat than the mind, and medical
research, to an overwhelming degree, has favored physical disease
rather than the emotional and behavioral difficulties of life. Compared with the U.S. estimate of 2.6% (Table 2.6), British findings
are that 10% of consultations in general practice are for mental
disorders (Office of Population Censuses and Surveys, 1974, Table
10). For the reasons mentioned above, the frequency of affective
problems in primary care in North America may be higher than
these statistics show.

Morbidity in community practice is a mixed picture, partly
predictable from mortality and disease frequency statistics but also
influenced by emotional, social, and demographic factors.

TABLE 2.6: Percent Distribution of Principal Diagnosis Categories in Office Visits to General and Family Practitioners, United States, January 1980 to December 1981

Principal Diagnosis Category	%
Diseases of the respiratory system	17.3
Diseases of the circulatory system	13.1
Injury & poisoning	9.8
Diseases of the musculoskeletal system & connective tissue	7.6
Endocrine, nutritional & metabolic diseases, immunity disorders	6.2
Diseases of the digestive system	5.6
Diseases of the genitourinary system	5.3
Diseases of the nervous system & sense organs	5.1
Diseases of the skin & subcutaneous tissue	4.0
Symptoms, signs & ill-defined conditions	3.8
Infections & parasitic diseases	3.3
Mental disorders	2.6
Neoplasms	1.2
Supplementary classification*	13.0
All other diagnoses	1.1
Unknown diagnoses	1.2

* Visits with no reported classifiable diagnosis or visits by persons who were not sick
Source: National Center for Health Statistics, 1983c, p. 28.

SUMMARY

The general health status of the population has been examined from a number of perspectives, each contributing a different dimension to the definition of the population's health. Mortality statistics have described health status in terms of death and loss of life, disease prevalence has defined the morbid problems with which individuals must live and cope, and a description of the quality of life has been provided by statistics of emotional and social health status. Institutional statistics serve to define the frequency with which people leave their own homes to reside in an institution. The demographic perspective has emphasized the importance of postponing the onset of chronic disease in an aging society and the need to examine the trends of disease occurrence. Finally, the profile of complaints in general practice has provided a definition of the health problems which the community perceives as being worthy of medical care. The uses of these various data are diverse. The frequency of diseases causing death and disability provide a general framework for research policy. Morbidity statistics, rather than mortality statistics, are of principal relevance to health services planning. Educational institutions that train clinicians require statistics on the frequency and nature of problems which are common in clinical practice. Statistics on utilization patterns and the diseases and illnesses presenting to hospitals and other health care institutions are essential to a rational policy for the organization of health care.

The focus of this chapter has been upon the health of the whole population and the development of an overview of health. This macroscopic view of the problem has a number of uses as listed above. However, such a general perspective has limitations. While the health of the total population might appear to be at an acceptable level, how can one detect if within the population there are not some people who are very much sicker and in need of more help than others? Summary statistics of the total population cannot single out subgroups in need. For example, if infant mortality is low does this mean that the poor, the geographically isolated, and immigrants all share an equally low risk of infant mortality? Commonly, the answer to this type of question is unknown.

Population health is often thought of as the study of health in the total population. If this was the limit of population health then the health of subgroups and populations at high risk would be overlooked. If health was distributed equally in society there would be no reasons to be concerned about groups within the total population. Unfortunately, the health of many groups in society is much worse than the average, and for this reason it is necessary to focus on these smaller populations which together make up the whole community.

Chapter 3

The Problem: The Health
of Specific Populations

Historically, the present high standard of health enjoyed by much of society is a recent development. Concurrent with this improvement has come a widening in the differences in health between various sectors of the population. Two or three centuries ago life expectancy for each stratum of society was probably quite similar.

In 17th century Europe a number of estimates of life expectancy indicated that the average length of life ranged between 24 and 34 years (Antonovsky, 1967, p. 32). At that time the low life expectancy tended to apply to all classes of society, including royalty (Hollingsworth, 1965). During the 18th century premature mortality started to decline and life expectancy began to improve. The improvements have favored certain sectors more than others. When life expectancy was barely sufficient to maintain survival of the race, there was little room for large differences to develop between groups. The unequalness which exists today between the health of various sectors of society has grown partly out of the different rates of improvement experienced during the 18th, 19th and 20th centuries. This is especially so for social class, racial, and regional differences. Differential health problems between various age groups and disease groups have probably arisen for other reasons.

The purpose of this chapter is to develop the concept of using specific populations as the focus for defining the health state of the community. As mentioned already, the relevance of this approach depends upon health problems being unequally distributed among different groups within society. Social class is one of the most important criteria for defining populations with specific health needs, but it is not the only one. Populations of interest defined by sociodemographic, geographic, and disease characteristics are also of current importance. The available data that distinguish demographic, cultural, and socioeconomic groups pertain mainly to mortality, whereas inequalities in morbidity are also relevant. Each of these broad categories of specific population will be considered in turn.

THE AMERICAN ELDERLY

Introduction

Among demographic variables, age is undoubtedly the most important; however, other variables such as sex, marital status, and parity also differentiate groups with particular health needs. Examples of age groups with specific problems include the elderly, who experience a wide spectrum of health problems; adolescent females with problems associated with reproduction; and males aged 15 to 25 years who experience a particularly high mortality due to accidents. There are many more examples, but let us now consider the health needs of the elderly.

Mortality

The relationship of age and mortality (Figure 2.1) is one in which death is progressively postponed to late in the life span. Death rates start to increase exponentially after the age of approximately 50 years, as shown by the age-specific death rates in Table 3.1. The risk of death by age 60 is two to three times that for the population as a whole, and by the age of 70 this rate has again doubled. A more precise picture is given by examining the specific causes of death.

Heart disease is the single most important contributor to mortality in the elderly; 1,144 of the 2,883 deaths per 100,000 in the 65 to 74 age group in 1983 were from this cause. For the same age group, 832 deaths per 100,000 were from cancer, of which 261 were respiratory in origin and 109 were cancer of the breast. Strokes accounted for 184 deaths per 100,000 in that age group. Motor vehicle accidents are also important contributors to death among the elderly. The death rate from road accidents in individuals 75 years of age and older is only surpassed by the rate among the 15 to 24-year-old age group. Perhaps of more concern than these accidents, because of associated morbidity, is that nearly as many elderly over the age of 75 die from suicide, and between

TABLE 3.1: Death Rates per 100,000 by Age for all Causes, United States, 1983

Age	Number of Deaths per 100,000 Resident Population (rounded to whole number)
Under 1 year	1,077
1 – 4 years	52
5 – 14 years	27
15 – 24 years	96
25 – 34 years	122
35 – 44 years	203
45 – 54 years	542
55 – 64 years	1,299
65 – 74 years	2,883
75 – 84 years	6,310
85 years and over	15,422

Source: National Center for Health Statistics, 1984d, p. 51.

the ages of 75 and 84 the suicide rate is higher than in any other age group (National Center for Health Statistics, 1984d, pp. 51–74).

Morbidity

The excessive health problems of the elderly are not limited to mortality. As illustrated in the Canada Health Survey the proportion of the elderly over 65 years who report at least one health problem is 86%, compared with 54% for the total population; and problems such as arthritis, rheumatism, hypertension, and heart disease are reported by the elderly at least four times as frequently as the population in general (Statistics Canada, 1981b, p. 115). Based on physical examination findings, between 1976 and 1980, 27% of noninstitutionalized Americans aged 65 to 74 had blood pressures above 160 mmHg systolic or 95 mmHg diastolic or both (National Center for Health Statistics, 1984d, p. 92). Service utilization rates reflect these findings. The annual rate of short-stay hospitalization in 1981 was 13% for individuals aged 65 and over, compared to 9% for the 45 to 64 years age group. Long-term institutionalization increases exponentially in the elderly (National Center for Health Statistics, 1981, p. 4; Wilkins and Adams, 1982). In the same year as the above, 1981, the number of physician visits per person was 6.3 for those aged 65 and over, while the average for all ages was 4.6 physician visits per year. A further measure of morbidity is disability days per person per year. The frequency of disability increases steadily with age. The elderly have twice as many disability and bed disability days per person as the average for all ages. Home accidents are overwhelmingly the most important cause of disability associated with the elderly. Limitation of activity in the elderly is associated with chronic disease more frequently than in younger individuals. The average rate of activity limitation from chronic disease is 14%, whereas in the elderly 46% of individuals with chronic disease experience limitation of activity due to their disorder (National Center for Health Statistics, 1982, pp. 20–30).

Discussion

Much of the disability and handicap of the elderly has resulted from the effect of degenerative diseases: arthritis, heart disease, pulmonary disease, and sensory loss. The underlying degenerative processes in these conditions are universal biological phenomena which begin in early life and progress incrementally. The process of degeneration advances more rapidly in some people than in others, due in part to behavior such as diet, smoking, and exercise. The ultimate onset of symptoms is also variable. The fortunate ones among us live their lives without restriction, while others experience painful immobility, hospitalization, and limitation in major activities (Fries & Crapo, 1981, pp. 79–95).

While death and biological degeneration are unavoidable, the impact of chronic disorders upon everyday life is potentially modifiable. Many physiological functions can be maintained at a level sufficient to support a disability-free life simply through continued use and training and avoiding certain abuses such as smoking and dietary excesses. These modifiable aspects of aging include cardiac and pulmonary reserve, memory and intelligence, bone density, physical strength and endurance, and social ability, among others (Fries & Crapo, 1981, p. 125). The unanswered questions are how much of the morbidity among the elderly can be avoided, and by what means. There is physiological evidence that much can be done to protect the health of our aging population (Fries & Crapo, 1981, pp. 107–132).

The elderly are a most important group to understand not only because of the very high prevalence of health problems among them, but also because of the growing size of the elderly population. For each male who reaches the age of 65 there is an average 14.5 years of life remaining, and females of the same age have 18.8

years of expected life yet to live (National Center for Health Statistics, 1984d, p. 53).

CULTURAL GROUPS

Health status also varies according to culture and ethnic origin. Among the many cultural groups in North America some stand out due to marked differences in health. Three groups will be used to illustrate the importance of giving specific attention to racial subpopulations; black and hispanic Americans and native Canadians.

Black Americans

Mortality among blacks at all ages exceeds death rates for whites. The age-specific death rates for black males in 1983 was 1,025 per 100,000. This compares unfavorably with the death rates in the same year for white males (702 per 100,000), black females (572 per 100,000), and white females (392 per 100,000). Life expectancy for blacks is correspondingly lower than for whites. For both sexes life expectancy at birth in 1983 was 69.6 years for blacks and 75.2 years for whites. The negative aspect of these figures is that inequalities in health between black and white Americans still exist. However, the situation has been far worse. In this century the differential in life expectancy between the two races has declined from 14.6 years in 1900 to 5.6 years in 1983. This favorable trend is continuing. Life expectancy at age 65, in comparison to life expectancy at birth, shows a smaller difference between races. Part of the explanation for this is the higher infant mortality rate among black Americans. In 1981 the black infant mortality rate was 20.0 per 1,000 live births, while among whites it was 10.5 per 1,000 live births. The situation is worse than this in some regions, such as in the east north central United States, where the black infant mortality rate was 23.8 per 1,000 live births in 1979–1981 (National Center for Health Statistics, 1984d, pp. 51–55).

All leading causes of death occur more frequently in blacks than whites (Table 3.2). Particularly notable are the high death rates among blacks from heart disease, strokes, malignancies, accidents, and homicide and legal intervention. The largest proportional difference between races is for maternal mortality. The death rate from complications of pregnancy, childbirth, and the puerperium was 22.1 per 100,000 live births among black women in 1981, compared with 6.5 per 100,000 live births in whites. Death rates from cancer of the breast are nearly the same in both races. Only motor vehicle death rates and suicide are lower in blacks than whites (National Center for Health Statistics, 1984d, pp. 59–76).

An important factor in the rate of heart disease and strokes is the occurrence of elevated blood pressure. High blood pressure in blacks is more frequent than in whites. Based on physical examinations of a sample of the civilian noninstitutionalized population aged 25–74, the prevalence of elevated blood pressure (systolic or diastolic pressure of at least 160 mmHg or diastolic pressure of at least 95 mmHg or both) in 1976–1980 was 1.4 times higher in black men than white men, and 2.3 times higher in black women than white women. During the same period, the frequency of elevated blood pressure was slightly greater in black women than black men, whereas white women had a moderately lower prevalence than white men. The prevalence of elevated blood pressure in blacks of both sexes combined was 24.6%. This is 8% lower than the frequency among blacks in 1960–1962 (National Center for Health Statistics, 1984d, p. 92).

TABLE 3.2: Age-Adjusted Death Rates per 100,000 for Selected Causes of Death, for Black and White Americans by Sex, 1981

Causes of Death	Death Rate (rounded)			
	Black		White	
	Male	Female	Male	Female
Heart disease	317	191	269	130
Cerebrovascular diseases	73	58	39	33
Malignant neoplasms	232	127	158	107
Respiratory system	84	20	58	19
Digestive system	62	35	39	25
Breast (female only)	—	24	—	23
Pneumonia and influenza	26	11	16	9
Chronic liver disease, cirrhosis	27	13	15	7
Diabetes mellitus	17	21	9	8
Accidents, adverse effects	75	22	59	20
Motor vehicle accidents	31	8	33	12
Suicide	11	3	19	6
Homicide, legal intervention	69	13	10	3

Source: National Center for Health Statistics, 1984d. pp. 59–60.

Discussion

Black Americans are unquestionably a subgroup of the population with special health needs beyond those of the average American. Maternal and infant health is one particular problem area. However, the health of blacks is improving continuously, and current black mortality rates generally correspond with those of the white population of approximately 20 years ago. The implication is that the health status of black Americans is modifiable through changing environmental factors. (This question is explored in detail in the following chapters.) An important exception, however, is the higher frequency of elevated blood pressure among blacks, for which there is no satisfactory explanation. The relatively low use of nursing homes among blacks suggests that black families provide more care for their elderly outside of institutions.

Morbidity Among Hispanic Americans

Hispanic races in the United States, including Mexican Americans, Puerto Ricans, Cuban Americans, and others, comprise another important racial subgroup. In this section, using various indicators of morbidity, the health of Hispanic Americans is compared with that of white and black Americans. These data come from National Health Survey interviews conducted in 1978, 1979, and 1980 (National Center for Health Statistics, 1984e).

Acute conditions, defined as illnesses and injuries that cause one or more days of restricted activity or medical attention, occur most frequently among whites, followed by Hispanic Americans, and occur least frequently among blacks. However, as Hispanic Americans are not homogeneous in their health status, it is more informative to describe the three major Hispanic subgroups separately. Puerto Ricans had the highest incidence of acute conditions, with an age-adjusted rate of 296 acute conditions per 100 persons per year. Whites had 229, and blacks, Mexican Americans, and Cuban Americans all had approximately 180 acute conditions per 100 persons per year. Puerto Ricans also had the highest frequency of restricted activity from injury or illness, and they spent the most time in bed for health reasons compared with other hispanic and nonhispanic persons. Specifically, Puerto Ricans reported 27 days of restricted activity per person per year, followed by blacks with 22 days per year. On average, Puerto Ricans spent 2 weeks in bed for health reasons and blacks had the second highest rate of bed days, with an average of 9 days per year.

Mexican Americans reported the lowest number of days of restricted activity among all Hispanic and nonhispanic groups. Long-term disability was assessed by the percentage of persons with activity limitation due to chronic conditions. The highest age-adjusted prevalence of limited activity from chronic conditions was among Puerto Ricans and blacks. Because the age composition of the Cuban American population is older than the other Hispanic groups, the crude rate of long-term disability was highest in Cuban Americans, whereas the age-adjusted rate is similar to other Hispanic groups and to white Americans (National Center for Health Statistics, 1984e, pp. 12–16, 43–44, 52).

Utilization of health services varied considerably among Hispanic groups. Mexican Americans averaged fewer visits to the physician, with 3.7 visits per person per year, than whites who had 4.8 visits and blacks who had 4.6 visits per year. Puerto Ricans and Cuban Americans averaged more visits, 6.0 and 6.2 visits per person per year respectively. These differences were independent of the age composition of the populations. Age-adjusted hospitalization rates were highest in Cuban Americans, of whom 12.2% were hospitalized once or more per year. The annual hospitalization rate was 11.5% among Puerto Ricans, 11.1% in blacks, and 10.3% in whites. The lowest rate was among Mexican Americans, of whom 9.6% were hospitalized per year (National Center for Health Statistics, 1984e, pp. 6–11). Nursing home occupancy also varies with race. The proportion of nonwhite Americans 65 years and over who were in nursing homes in 1977 was 30 per 1,000, compared with 50 per 1,000 whites (National Center for Health Statistics, 1984d, p. 116).

Discussion

In summary, parameters of health of Hispanic Americans range from being inferior to the health status of blacks and whites, in the case of Puerto Ricans, to being superior to blacks and whites, in the case of Mexican Americans. The health of Puerto Ricans was observed to be worse than the rest of the population in terms of the occurrence of acute conditions, restriction of activity from illness and injury, and from long-term disability. Mexican Americans, on the other hand, tended to be among the healthiest in the population in terms of these parameters. Concerning health utilization, Cuban Americans and Puerto Ricans had the highest rates, whereas Mexican Americans had rates lower than all other racial groups.

These findings cannot be explained simply. It is well recognized that the frequency of acute conditions, disability, and service utilization relate to a number of attributes including age, sex, income, educational level, and perceived health status (National Center for Health Statistics, 1984e, pp. 6-16). The distribution of these or other attributes within the Hispanic groups may explain some or all of the observed differences. Sampling error is also a possible explanation. Finally, it may be that the health status of Hispanic Americans is truly diverse, so that the health of some Hispanic groups is worse than that of the average American and others are in fact better. More information needs to be acquired before we fully understand the health of these racial minorities.

The Canadian Native Population

We will move now to the north of the continent and describe the health of Canadian Native Indians and Inuit (Eskimos).

The 312,430 native Indians in Canada are distributed across all regions, although only 1% live in the Yukon and 2.5% in the North West Territories (NWT). The Inuit, on the other hand, reside in the far north; 15,650 in the NWT, 4,950 in Quebec (Health and Welfare, Canada, 1982, pp,. 37-38), and less than 5,000 distributed across all other provinces (Statistics Canada, 1983b, pp. 6-7).

In 1981 life expectancy among the native Indian population was 62 years for males and 69 years for females (Rowe and Norris, 1985, p. 65), which is nearly a decade less than the Canadian average. The crude mortality rates (CDR) do not reflect this difference. In 1980 the CDR for Indians was 5.9 per 1,000 per year, compared with 7.2 per 1,000 per year for the total population (Health and Welfare Canada, 1983, p. 35; Statistics Canada, 1982b, p. 46). This apparent discrepancy is due to the younger age composition of the native population. It is therefore useful to consider the deaths in each age group separately. All death rates up to late middle age are higher in the Indian than in the total population. This difference is greatest among infants, children, and young adults between 25 and 34 years of age. The difference in infant mortality is mainly due to an approximately three times higher postneonatal mortality rate among Indians than in the total population (Health and Welfare Canada, 1983, pp. 35, 37; Statistics Canada, 1982b, p. 2).

The higher rates of premature death among the native population would suggest that the relative importance in certain causes of death may also differ. This is the case as shown in Table 3.3 Deaths from accidents, poisoning, and violence are the leading causes of mortality for both Indians and Inuit. Among the Indians deaths from these causes exceed by three times the rate for the whole population. The situation is reversed for vascular disease deaths. Both Indians and Inuit have less than half the rate of circulatory system deaths of other Canadians. Respiratory disease deaths are a major problem for the Inuit; their death rate from these diseases is twice that for both Indians and the general population. Suicides are high in both native groups between 15 and 40 years of age. Indian suicide rates for 1980 were highest between the ages of 25 and 29, for which the rate was 112 per 100,000 per year, compared with 33 per 100,000 for male Canadians of the same age (Health and Welfare Canada, 1982, pp. 9–10, 47; Statistics Canada, 1982a, p. 24).

While systematic morbidity data on the total native population are not available, a survey of Indians in Northwestern Ontario (Young, 1979a, p. 215) found respiratory infections to be the most common problem in ambulatory care, followed by skin infections and trauma.

Discussion

The health of natives in terms of life expectancy and premature mortality is a great deal worse than that experienced by other Canadians. The high rates of infection, trauma, and postneonatal morbidity and mortality describe a distinctive pattern of illness. Underlying these problems are a multitude of factors which together are peculiar to the native population. Much of their cultural inheritance has been changed and lost. Assimilation into western society is only partial. The result is a state of being between two ways of life and divided between two distinct sets of cultural

TABLE 3.3: Death Rates per 100,000 for Leading Causes of Death, Canadian Indian and Inuit, 1980

Causes of Death	Indian	Inuit	Canada (1979)
Accidents	239.3	159.7	70.0
Circulatory system	144.7	159.7	335.9
Respiratory system	50.9	108.6	43.4

Source: Health and Welfare Canada, 1982, p. 9.

values and beliefs. In many instances resources for an independent existence are lacking, and a sense of control over one's life is diminished. The native population has become handicapped in its ability to lead a full and satisfying life. It is not surprising that emotional health is affected; this is reflected in the high suicide rate and the frequency of violence and alcoholism.

The Canadian native population is therefore a special group which needs to be understood in terms of both its particular health problems and the underlying cultural, economic, psychological, social, and political circumstances which accompany these problems. Although natives have been referred to as one group, this is an oversimplification. Some Indians live and work in southern Canada with few of the environmental disadvantages of those in the north. The health of these southern Indians tends to match that of other Canadians rather than that of other natives. An accurate appraisal therefore requires an analysis at a level where there is an appropriate degree of homogeneity in terms of the social environment as well as ethnicity.

THE POOR IN CANADA

Introduction

The problem of inequalities in health between the poor and the rest of society has many manifestations. The general nature of these differences is graphically illustrated by health conditions in 19th century England. John Snow in his classic account of cholera wrote:

> Mr. Baker, of Staines, who attended two hundred and sixty cases of cholera and diarrhea in 1849, chiefly among the poor, informed me in a letter with which he favoured me in December of that year, that 'when the patients passed their stools involuntarily the disease evidently spread.' It is amongst the poor, where a whole family live, sleep, cook, eat and wash in a single room, that cholera has been found to spread when once introduced, and still more in those places termed common lodging houses, in which several families were crowded into a single room. It was amongst the vagrant class, who lived in this crowded state, that cholera was most fatal in 1832; but the Act of Parliament for the regulation of common lodging-houses, has caused the disease to be much less fatal amongst these people in the late epidemics. When, on the other hand, cholera is introduced into the better kind

of houses, as it often is . . . it hardly ever spreads from one member of the family to another. The constant use of the hand-basin and towel, and the fact of the apartments for cooking and eating being distinct from the sick room, are the cause of this. (Snow, 1936, p. 18)

During the approximately 130 years since the time of Snow's writing the problem of cholera has disappeared, but major differences in health between the rich and poor continue to exist.

Life Expectancy

The majority of Canadian data on life expectancy and mortality come from Wigle and Mao's (1980) work on mortality by income level in urban Canada. In their analysis the level of income was defined using the median household income of the census tract of residence based on the 1971 Census of Canada, and it was categorized according to the following five income levels: $11,456 or more; $9,686-$11,455; $8,543-$9,685; $7,391-$8,542; and $7,390 or less. The population included in their study accounted for 54% of the total for Canada in 1971 (Wigle & Mao, 1980, pp. 22-23).

Despite the overall prosperity of Canada, there are readily identifiable differences in life expectancy between income categories. In 1971 female life expectancy ranged from 74.6 years in income level 5 to 77.5 in level 1. For men the difference in life expectancy between the highest and lowest income level was 6.2 years. Men in level 5 had a life expectancy of 66.3 years, compared with 72.5 years in the top income level (Wigle & Mao, 1980, pp. 8, 27). Although life expectancy is continuing to improve, albeit by small increments, the situation for level 5 males is quite unfavorable. Based on a conservative calculation, Wilkins (1980a, p. 22) had estimated that mortality for males in level 5 in 1974 was at least as high or higher than that experienced by the average Canadian male a generation earlier. In a study of differential mortality in Montreal from 1961 to 1976, the same author (Wilkins, 1980b, p. 9) found that the 9-year disparity in life expectancy between the highest and lowest income levels of the city had not diminished during this 15-year period.

Mortality

The pattern of mortality across income levels is described in Table 3.4. The age-standardized death rate ranges from 7.2 per 1,000 per year for level 1 males to 10.67 for level 5 males; for females a gradient also exists, but it is of a smaller magnitude. The largest difference between male and female mortality is in level 5, where the male/female mortality ratio is 2 (Wigle & Mao, 1980, p. 28).

When mortality is examined by both sex and age, a gradient is apparent between income levels in nearly all age–sex groups as shown in Table 3.5. This table displays comparative mortality figures (CMF) by age and sex. A CMF is the ratio of two age-adjusted death rates. In this case the denominator is the death rate for income level 1. The CMF is the same as a standardized mortality ratio (SMR) and is interpreted similarly (see Chapter 2, "Methodology"). It expresses the relative difference in mortality between two groups. The largest relative difference between income levels occurs in infants of both sexes, male children 1 to 14 years of age, and in males between the ages of 35 and 64. The gradient is smallest in elderly males and is not apparent among women over 65 (Wigle & Mao, 1980, p. 28).

The CMF does not indicate absolute differences in mortality. Where death rates are very high a modest CMF can be based on large absolute differences in mortality. For example, the CMF for income level 5 males over 65 years is 127; this is based on an absolute difference in mortality between income levels 1 and 5 of 1,548 deaths per 100,000 per year. Other large absolute differences in age-specific death rates between income levels 1 and 5 are 1,173 per 100,000 per year for male infants, 855 for female infants, and 591 for males 35 to 64 years (Wigle & Mao, 1980, p. 21).

When death rates are examined by cause of death, the same gradient with income is found. Table 3.6 displays the age-standardized death rates for selected causes of death. The largest difference in death rates between high and low income levels is

TABLE 3.4: Age-Adjusted Death Rates per 1,000 by Income Level and Sex, Canada, 1971

	Income Level	Males	Females	Ratio M/F
1	High	7.20	4.35	1.66
2		7.82	4.43	1.77
3		8.48	4.73	1.79
4		8.87	5.05	1.76
5	Low	10.67	5.32	2.01
Ratio 5/1		1.48	1.22	

Source: Wigle DI and Mao Y. 1980, p. 28.

TABLE 3.5: Comparative Mortality Figures* (using income level 1 as reference) by age, sex, and income level, Canada, 1971

		Income Level				
Age	Sex	1	2	3	4	5
Infants	M	100	121	145	162	195
	F	100	115	125	145	187
Children	M	100	145	136	187	194
1 – 14	F	100	106	112	134	151
Adults	M	100	110	129	126	149
15 – 34	F	100	111	123	137	152
Adults	M	100	114	129	141	193
35 – 64	F	100	109	110	131	151
Elderly	M	100	105	111	112	127
65 and over	F	100	98	107	107	105

* See text for definition.
Source: Wigle DT, and Mao Y. 1980, p. 28.

TABLE 3.6: Age-Adjusted death rates per 100,000 by cause, sex, and income level, Canada, 1971

	Female Income Levels		Males Income Levels	
Cause of Death	High	Low	High	Low
All causes	435	532	720	1067
Circulatory system	209	239	371	492
Neoplasms	118	126	160	214
Accidents, poisonings, violence	31	45	59	111
Respiratory system	19	27	41	83
Digestive system	14	24	24	52
Other causes	44	71	65	115

Source: Wigle DT and Mao T. 1980, p. 21.

for male circulatory system deaths. Next in order are male deaths from neoplasms, accidents, and respiratory disease (Wigle & Mao, 1980, p. 21).

Given the increasing incidence of most of these diseases with age, it is to be expected that the largest absolute differences in mortality for each cause would occur in the elderly. First, consider circulatory disease. The difference in age-specific death rates (ASDRs) between the high and low income levels for males 65 years and over is 721 deaths per 100,000 per year. The difference in ASDRs for males aged 35 to 64 is 201, and for females aged 65 and over it is 103. In the case of neoplasms the ASDR difference between high and low income levels is 271 for males over 65 and 100 for males aged 35 to 64. By contrast, in the case of respiratory deaths an important component of the difference between income level is infant mortality. The ASDR difference between high and low income levels is 256 for males over 65, 158 for female infants, 108 for male infants, and 59 for males aged 35 to 64. For diseases of the digestive system the difference is greater for males over 65 years, 110 deaths per 100,000 per year; and for males aged 35 to 64, it is 65 (Wigle & Mao, 1980, p. 21).

In addition to these general disease categories, there are some specific causes of death for which the relative difference in mortality between income levels is considerable. The first of these is death from tuberculosis in income level 5, for which the CMF for males is 1,361 and for females is 528. The CMF for income level 5 for deaths due to pregnancy, childbirth, and during the puerperium is 339. Finally, in the case of lung cancer the CMF for income level 5 is 234 for males (Wigle & Mao, 1980, pp. 19, 30).

The current situation concerning mortality is clearly one in which the lower socioeconomic groups have significantly poorer health than the higher income groups. Given this inequity it is important to ask whether the situation is changing. To respond to the question it is helpful to refer to the Black Report (Townsend & Davidson, 1982) from the United Kingdom, which is one of the most extensive works on health and social class (defined by occupation). Between 1949 and 1972 in Britain the mortality rate declined among most occupational classes but not in all age-sex groups. Men aged 55 to 64 in the low occupational groups experienced an increase in mortality, and for other men and women aged between 45 and 64 in the low occupational groups there was little or no improvement in mortality. The decline in death rates during this period was greatest among the upper social classes and the young. The effect of large improvements in mortality among the upper classes, combined with a small or negative change among older age groups in the lower classes, has increased the difference in health status between social classes (Townsend & Davidson, 1982, p. 68).

Morbidity

The pattern of inequality between social classes does not stop with mortality. Lower socioeconomic groups also have a significantly higher level of morbidity and hospital usage. Approximately 33% of all mental disorders, heart disease, bronchitis and emphysema, and sight problems were reported in the 20% of the Canadian population with the lowest income. The frequency of these problems declines as income increases. Negative affect and symptoms of anxiety and depression were also found to be more frequent among low income groups (Statistics Canada, 1981b, pp. 117, 137).

It would be expected that with higher rates of health problems the lower income groups would make more use of health services. This is mostly the case. The situation in Britain is that general practitioner attendance and hospital usage is higher for lower socioeconomic groups than it is for others. In contrast, however, attendance at preventive services such as antenatal clinics is lower for poor classes than for the more prosperous (Townsend & Davidson, 1982, pp. 76–89).

Discussion

In this section it has been shown that lower socioeconomic groups experience an excess of the national burden of ill health. This affects utilization of health services and frequency of disease as well as death rates and life expectancy. There are indications that for at least some groups the situation is not improving. Lower social class is not uniformly associated with bad health; for example, females are not as affected as males and health differences are more marked in certain age groups. Discrepancies are greatest in infants and children. Some of the major problems include excessive respiratory disease in lower income male and female infants, an excess of accidents in lower income male children, and an increased incidence of heart disease, cancer, accidents, and respiratory disease among low income middle-aged males.

The issues raised by these problems concern understanding why these differences exist, and finding methods to improve the health of the poor. Consideration should first be given to the possibility of these findings being invalid due to bias in the selection of subjects, measurement of variables, or in the analysis of data. A thorough appraisal of these methodological issues has resulted in the possibility of such methodological inaccuracy being refuted (Townsend & Davidson, 1982, p. 113). The three remaining categories of possible explanation for the aggregation of health problems among the poor are that: (1) low socioeconomic status is a cause of poor health; (2) poor health itself is responsible for low socioeconomic status; and (3) some "third" factor other than socioeconomic status of poor health is responsible. There is no clear answer as to which explanation(s) applies. The first and third explanations will be explored in subsequent chapters. A factor of importance is that health-related behavior such as smoking varies across social classes. These and other aspects of life-style will be examined in terms of their contribution to health and illness in Chapters 5 and 6.

GROUPS WITH SPECIFIC HEALTH PROBLEMS

Introduction

In this section a different type of population is described. In contrast to defining a population by demographic criteria such as economic status, age, or race, the focus will be upon populations defined according to specific health problems. While disease groups are the commonest type of specific population studied in biomedical and therapeutic research, populations of stroke patients, heart disease patients, or paraplegics, for example, are studied relatively uncommonly for purposes of understanding the problems outside the biological disease process which affect how patients live their lives. Consequently, there is comparatively little scientific description of the general health needs of specific disease groups. Epidemiological studies are needed to describe the natural history of the consequences of disease upon everyday life as well as the biological course of disease. The focus of epidemiological research has tended to be in areas other than the behavioral consequences of disease. The orientation has been predominantly on antecedents to disease and on the biological events which characterize its course, while clinical epidemiology has developed primarily around the investigation of therapeutic strategies designed to alter the biological course of disease. Consequently, our understanding of the impairment, disability, and handicap associated with chronic disease is limited. Research is needed to define the magnitude of these problems, to describe their distribution, to expand our understanding of their etiology, and to find effective strategies for their care and management.

The Consequences of Disease

As mentioned in Chapter 1, the International Classification of Impairments, Disabilities and Handicaps developed by the World Health Organization (1980) is a taxonomy of the consequences of disease. The stages in the clinical progression of chronic disease provide the framework for the classification. When a chronic disease occurs, the initial phase in the process is development of pathological changes in tissues which manifest themselves as clinical signs or symptoms. This is the level of focus of the medical model of disease. Beyond this are three levels of consequences. An early consequence of disease is the realization that the individual is unwell due to impairment at the level of a body organ. This may or may not lead to disability or alteration in individual performance and subsequently to some degree of handicap in social role.

Impairment refers to deviation from a biomedical norm at an organ level. As such it is any loss or abnormality of psychological, physiological, or anatomical structure or function. Some major categories of impairment include intellectual, language, other psychological, aural, ocular, visceral, skeletal, and disfiguring impairments (World Health Organization, 1980, p. 27).

Disability in the health context is any restriction or lack (resulting from impairment) of ability to perform an activity in a normal manner. Disability is concerned with integrated activities at the level of the whole person such as communication, personal care, locomotion, and dexterity, among others (World Health Organization, 1980, p. 28).

Handicap, which results from impairment or disability, is a limitation in the fulfillment of a role that is normal for the given individual. This may take the form of a handicap in orientation, physical independence, mobility, occupation, social integration, economic self-sufficiency, and others (World Health Organization, 1980, p. 29).

Populations with specific health problems may be defined either by their handicap or the underlying disease. As an illustration one population of each type will be described.

The physically handicapped in Ontario not residing in institutions were surveyed in 1980 (Ministry of Health, 1982) by taking a stratified sample of 15,948 households. From this, 1,764 physically handicapped respondents were identified who were estimated to be 73% of all individuals with a physical handicap in the sampled dwellings. This group completed the "Physical and Health Problems in the Household" questionnaire which had been mailed to them. Even though the prevalence of physical handicap increases with age a moderate proportion of the physically handicapped in this survey were relatively young. Nineteen percent were under 40 years of age and 35% were between the ages of 40 and 59. Economically they are a disadvantaged group, 40% having a family income under $5,000 per annum (Ministry of Health, 1982, pp. 16, 24).

Thirty-two percent had a musculoskeletal impairment, and cardiovascular and neurological impairment affected 25% and 10% respectively. Table 3.7 shows the frequency of various disabilities and handicaps. Those affecting social integration, mobility, economic self-sufficiency, and occupation were all prevalent, while difficulty and limitation with recreation and social activity was the most frequent handicap (Ministry of Health, 1982, pp. 30, 46).

A population such as the noninstitutionalized physically handicapped is heterogeneous in terms of the disease types it includes. When the purpose of a study is to define the social impact of disease in general, it is preferable to survey directly the prevalence of handicap in the total population, as was the case with this study of physically handicapped persons. Conversely, investigations of specific disease groups are necessary in order to develop knowledge and understanding of the natural history of disability and handicap among patients with given diseases. This is important for clinical practice. With the growing interest in quality of life more investigations into the consequences of diseases are being conducted, including those of specific disease groups. One such example is the study of multiple sclerosis.

Multiple sclerosis (MS) is but one chronic disorder with a high level of associated handicap and disability. The importance of

TABLE 3.7: Prevalence of Specific Types of Disability and Handicap Among the Noninstitutional Physically Handicapped in Ontario, 1980

Disabilities/Handicaps	Prevalence (%)
Recreation/social activities	20
Day to day functioning	18
Entry/exit from buildings	14
Income security	14
Finding a job	13
Mobility in community	11
Transportation	11

Source: Ministry of Health, 1982, p. 46.

developing an understanding of the social impact of this disease is increased by the lack of a cure or effective treatment of the disease itself. Prevalence studies provide a definition of the problem, describing the magnitude of the associated social morbidity. Prospective studies are needed to investigate prognosis, the course of associated disability, and treatment of difficulties in everyday living.

Among the impairments caused by MS the physical manifestations of the disease have been studied most extensively. The prevalence of specific neurological signs has been well described (Shepherd, 1979), and much work has been done in assessing disease severity (Kurtzke, 1970). Some studies have investigated the prevalence of psychological impairment in MS, which has been found to range between 39% in a U.S. study (Dalos et al., 1983) and 46% in a Canadian survey (Harper et al., 1986). Psychological impairment during periods when the disease is stable does not appear to correlate with disease severity (Dalos et al., 1983; Harper et al., 1986).

In a study in Ottawa, personal care disability and ambulation disability have been estimated to have a prevalence of 42% and 75%, respectively (Bennett et al., 1977). These forms of disability correlate closely with disease severity (Harper et al., 1986). Occupation handicap has been found to have a prevalence of 56% in a substantially disabled English group of MS patients (Elian & Dean, 1983). Among noninstitutionalized MS patients, social integration handicap was found to have a 28% prevalence rate and was only loosely related to disease severity. These rates far exceed those in the general population and in family practice patients in general (Harper et al., 1986). Psychological impairment in MS patients exceeds that in spinal cord injury patients by a factor of three (Dalos et al., 1983).

In addition to these specific problems of disability and handicap there is the added obstacle of public attitude towards disabled persons. The nondisabled members of society have been accused of disregarding the needs of disabled persons in many ways, including the protection of human and civil rights and the planning of health care services, employment, housing, shopping, education, recreation, communication, and transportation (Smith, 1981a, p. 4).

SUMMARY

In the midst of society's enthusiasm for preventing illness and promoting health it is enticing to overlook the individuals who are already disabled and ill. The numerous members of society whose disability cannot be cured need to adjust themselves to the permanent reality of impairment disability and handicap. The high standard of health enjoyed by the majority of North Americans, and western society in general, will overshadow the illness of minorities if we do not examine separately the health of specific sectors of society. In this chapter a few examples have illustrated how the health of the elderly, black Americans, Puerto Ricans, Canadian Natives, the poor, and the physically disabled all have special needs which are far greater than the average member of society. Inequalities in health present a particularly challenging and current problem to the health care system. While some inequalities are diminishing, others are not, and the difference in health status between the healthy and some high risk groups may be widening. Meeting the health needs of these specific sectors will require inquiry and investigation that are sensitive to the individual characteristics of these groups and that will therefore look beyond the encouraging picture demonstrated by national health statistics to the problem spots concealed within.

Chapter 4

Risks I: Concepts and Methods

In the preceding two chapters health problems have been described in terms of their diversity and distribution. Within this general picture considerable inequality exists in the distribution of disease and illness among the various sectors of society. Significantly higher frequency rates occur in groups such as the elderly, the poor, native groups, males, and the young. While description of the prevalence and distribution of health problems does not explain their occurrence, these empirical data do provide a scientific basis for the development of questions and hypotheses concerning possible mechanisms of predisposition and etiology.

This chapter and the two chapters that follow deal with the causes of disease and illness. As currently understood the causation of modern day disease is complex and multifactorial. To introduce the present situation and to develop a general conceptual framework of risk and causation the first half of this chapter is devoted to an historical analysis of health. This analysis identifies the diverse nature of factors affecting health and the change in the role of various factors from one time period to another. The second half of the chapter deals first with the concepts of risk, causation, and prognosis, and then with the methodological aspects of data concerning etiology and the natural history of disease.

McKEOWN'S HISTORICAL PERSPECTIVE

Examination of past patterns of health through a historical perspective is one approach to understanding current problems. This general approach provides a framework for more detailed inquiry.

The most notable analysis of this kind is the work of Thomas McKeown (1976, 1979). In his classic study of the decline in mortality in England and Wales from the 18th century to the present, McKeown has anlayzed causes of death in terms of the possible factors leading to the increase in life expectancy. Through this analysis he identifies the major determinants of health, including the role of medicine as one determinant.

For nearly three centuries the world population has been undergoing unprecedented changes. Although fluctuations in population size have occurred at previous times none have been as big or as sustained as the present exponential increase. At the time of William the Conquerer the population of England and Wales was estimated at 1.5 million. It increased only gradually over the next 6½ centuries, and the population in 1700 was 5.5 million. By 1971 it was almost 50 million (McKeown, 1976, p.1).

Accompanying the modern rise in population has been a dramatic increase in life expectancy and a comparable fall in mortality. While there exist other relevant indicators of improvement in health, life expectancy and mortality are particularly important. Therefore if priority is to be allocated among a variety of health promoting strategies, all of which are beneficial, it is necessary to know which ones influence the death rate and life expectancy. For this reason it is important to identify the factors responsible for the decline in mortality.

Although national statistics on the causes of death in England and Wales were not available until 1838 (start of registration of causes of death) the growth in population during the preceding century is sufficient reason to attempt an analysis of mortality from 1700. In Table 4.1 the reduction in mortality is shown for three periods: 1700 to the mid-19th century (a third); the second half of the 19th century (a fifth); and the 20th century (nearly half). These data are based on the assumption that the death rate in England and Wales in 1700 was 30 per 1,000 per year (McKeown, 1979, pp. 30–31).

Causes of Death 1848 to 1971

Despite the uncertain accuracy of statistics on the cause of death something can be learned from the examination of these data. In the following analysis conditions attributable to microorganisms are distinguished from conditions which are not. It is recognized that this distinction cannot be made in all cases, but generally

TABLE 4.1: Reduction of Mortality Since 1700: England and Wales

Period	% of total reduction in each period*	% of reduction due to infections
1700 to 1848–1854	33	?
1848–1854 to 1901	20	92
1901 to 1971	47	73
1700 to 1971	100	

* The estimates are based on the assumption that the death rate in 1700 was 30.
From T. McKeown, *The Role of Medicine: Dream, Mirage or Nemesis?*, p. 31. Copyright © 1979 by Princeton University Press. Reprinted by permission of Princeton University Press and Basil Blackwell, Ltd., Oxford, England.

this broad grouping can be made with reasonable confidence (McKeown, 1979, pp. 32–33).

The death rate in 1848–1854, 21,856 per million per year, was reduced to approximately one-fourth this size by 1971, 5,384 per million per year. Infectious diseases accounted for 59% of all deaths in 1848–1854, whereas only 13% of deaths in 1971 were due to microorganisms. Mortality in 1971 from infections was only 6% of the 1848–1854 rate of 12,965 per million per year. These were not the only diseases to decline. In addition, deaths due to noninfectious causes were approximately halved during this period. [See Figure 4.1 (McKeown, 1979, pp. 34–40).]

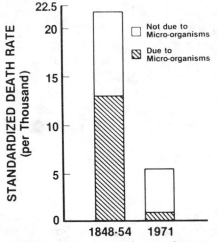

FIGURE 4–1 Mortality from infective and noninfective causes, 1848–1854 and 1971, England and Wales (Data from McKeown, 1979, pp. 34–39).

In Table 4.2 the estimates of the reduction in mortality from infectious causes are divided into three groups: airborne; water- and food-borne; and other. Airborne diseases were responsible for 40% of the reduction since the mid-19th century, compared with 21% from water- and food-borne diseases and 13% from other infections. Noninfectious conditions accounted for 26% of the decline in mortality (McKeown, 1979, pp. 33–34).

Respiratory tuberculosis was not only the most important airborne disease, but being responsible for 17.5% of mortality reduction from all causes, it accounts for a greater proportion of the decline in mortality than any other single disease. More than half of this decline occurred before the end of the 19th century. The group of bronchitis, pneumonia, and influenza was the second largest contributor of the airborne diseases, accounting for 9.9% of the reduction in mortality. Although most of this improvement was in the 20th century there is evidence that it started prior to the turn of the century. Diphtheria and scarlet fever accounted for 6.2% of the fall in mortality, three-fifths of which occurred before 1901. Whooping cough and measles made some contribution to the decline in mortality, mainly after 1901. Almost all of the 1.6% of the reduction due to smallpox occurred before 1901 (McKeown, 1979, pp. 34–35).

Nearly 50% of the reduction in mortality contributed by cholera, diarrhea, dysentery, nonrespiratory tuberculosis, typhoid, and typhus occurred before 1901. It is important to note that the rate

TABLE 4.2: Reduction of mortality for infectious and noninfectious diseases, 1848–1854 to 1971: England and Wales

Conditions Attributable to Microorganisms	% of Reduction
Airborne diseases	40
Water- and food-borne diseases	21
Other conditions	13
Total	74
Conditions not attributable to microorganisms	26
All diseases	100

The estimate of the proportion of deaths associated with microorganisms is lower than would be suggested in Table 4.1, because when the whole period (1848–1854 to 1971) is considered, certain infections (for example, rheumatic fever) cannot be included.

From T. McKeown, *The Role of Medicine: Dream, Mirage or Nemesis?*, p. 33. Copyright © 1979 by Princeton University Press. Reprinted by permission of Princeton University Press and Basil Blackwell, Ltd., Oxford, England.

of decline in mortality before 1901 was much greater for water-borne enteric diseases than for diarrheal diseases spread mainly by food (McKeown, 1979, pp. 35–37).

The noninfective diseases are a heterogeneous mixture, the study of which is limited by problems in classification. Of the 26% of the reduction in mortality since 1848–1854 contributed by non-infective diseases, nine-tenths occurred after the turn of the century. While the mortality from noninfectious causes in general experienced a decline from 8,891 deaths in 1848–1854 to 4,670 deaths per million per year in 1971, there are three categories of disease for which mortality has increased. (See Table 4.3) The increases in death due to myocardial infarction and lung cancer this century are primarily responsible for the overall increase in cardiovascular and cancer mortality. These increases overshadow concurrent declines in other forms of cardiovascular and malignant diseases. The decline in noninfectious causes of mortality was greater for females than males; this means that the reduction in overall noninfective mortality for male nonsmokers is underesti-mated (McKeown, 1979, pp. 38–40).

Causes of Death 1700 to 1848

During this period there is no convincing evidence concerning individual diseases; consequently inferences need to be based on subsequent events. From 1838 on, the airborne diseases, and particularly respiratory tuberculosis, were declining rapidly. Tu-berculosis was responsible for nearly half the total decline in deaths during the second half of the 19th century. During the 17th and 18th centuries mortality from tuberculosis was consid-erable, and given its decline at the time of first registration of causes of death it may have been falling earlier. Smallpox most probably declined during the preregistration period; by 1848–1854, its death rate was low (263 per million per year) relative to

TABLE 4.3: Standardized death rates per million from diseases which increased between 1848–1854 and 1971: England and Wales

Cause	1848–1854	1971
Cardiovascular disease	698	1,776
Cancer	307	1,169
Congenital defects	28	127

Source: Data from McKeown, 1979, p. 39.

respiratory tuberculosis, whooping cough, and measles. There is less certainty about the other airborne diseases. Similarly, there is a paucity of evidence concerning water- and food-borne diseases. During the postregistration period these diseases did not decline until there were improvements in water supply and sewage disposal starting in the 1870's. Prior to this, the growth in population, industrial development, and urbanization would have increased exposure to water-and food-borne disease. The appearance of cholera in England prior to registration, possibly for the first time, indicates a deterioration in hygiene. For these reasons it is most probable that the decline in mortality prior to 1848 was due to reduction of deaths from infectious diseases. The possible exceptions to this are reductions due to decline in deaths from starvation and infanticide. There is little convincing evidence that noninfectious causes of death declined between 1848–1854 and 1901 (McKeown, 1979, pp. 40–44).

Framework of Analysis

Having proposed that a reduction in infectious disease deaths was the prime reason for the decline in mortality, it is paradoxical that during this period the modern agricultural and industrial revolutions led to an aggregation of larger and denser populations than had ever existed previously. In searching for an explanation to the decline in mortality, it is important to examine the characteristics of microorganisms, the conditions under which they spread, and the response of the human host. Microorganisms and the host should not be considered separately; both are living organisms interacting with one another. When analyzing the role of the major influences on the infectious diseases, it is therefore necessary to distinguish between the following four factors.

1. *Interaction between organism and host.* Exposure to microorganisms over a period of time can lead to a genetically determined form of resistance. Immunity can also be acquired. Neither form of immunity is due to medical intervention or to identifiable environmental factors.

2. *Immunization and therapy.* Immunity may result from effective immunization and the outcome of infection can be influenced by therapy.

3. *Modes of spread.* The mode of spread of infection differs with the microorganism, and prevention depends largely upon interruption of transmission.

4. *The nutritional state of the host.* In addition to immunity, the host's state of health and nutrition influences the effect of exposure to microorganisms.

This classification is the basis for the following analysis of the reasons for the decline in mortality from infectious diseases (McKeown, 1979, pp. 45–46).

If a change in the character of the airborne diseases accounts for their decline, either one of the following two explanations would need to apply. First, there would need to have been a major reduction in virulence of all airborne infections similar to that which has occurred with scarlet fever (McKeown, 1976, pp. 82–83). In the light of the extent and duration of the fall in mortality, this explanation is untenable. Second, there would need to have been certain deleterious influences leading to high mortality in the 18th century that through natural selection resulted in survival of more resistant populations. Since there is no evidence of a large increase in mortality from infectious disease during the 18th century—in fact, indirect evidence suggests a decline—this explanation is also unacceptable. While some alteration in the nature of the infectious diseases probably occurred this was likely to have been insufficient to result in the substantial decline in mortality (McKeown, 1979, pp. 46–50).

The airborne diseases are the most important to consider in respect to immunization and therapy because of the magnitude of the decline in mortality attributed to them and because there is an obvious alternate explanation for the decline in water- and food-borne infections. The general pattern of the relation between the decline in mortality from airborne diseases and medical measures is illustrated in Figure 4.2, showing death rates from respiratory tuberculosis. Mortality from this disease had dropped from 4,000 to below 2,000 per million per year before the tubercle bacillus was identified. Mortality was below 500 per million per year before chemotherapy and Bacillus Calmette-Guérin (BCG) vaccination were introduced. Surgical treatment employed during the first half of this century was of little value (McKeown, 1979, pp. 50, 52).

In Table 4.4 are displayed the declines in mortality since the introduction of specific measures of prophylaxis and treatment for

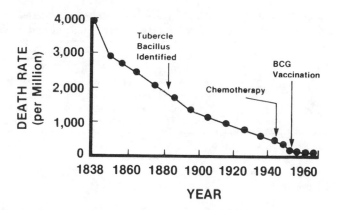

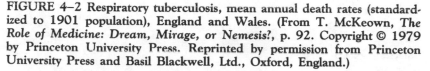

FIGURE 4-2 Respiratory tuberculosis, mean annual death rates (standardized to 1901 population), England and Wales. (From T. McKeown, *The
Role of Medicine: Dream, Mirage, or Nemesis?*, p. 92. Copyright © 1979
by Princeton University Press. Reprinted by permission from Princeton
University Press and Basil Blackwell, Ltd., Oxford, England.)

all major airborne infections. In the case of bronchitis, pneumonia,
and influenza, specific measures were ineffective prior to the introduction of sulphonamides in 1938. Since then 32% of the
reduction in deaths due to these diseases has occurred. The
majority of the decline in deaths from whooping cough and measles
preceded medical therapy. There was no effective treatment for
scarlet fever before sulphonamides became available. Diphtheria
antitoxin, introduced in 1894, is considered to have had a beneficial
effect on both case fatality and incidence. Smallpox vaccine, which
was first used in 1798, is generally considered responsible for the
eradication of the disease. Mortality was declining before, and
mostly long before, the introduction of effective measures, and
the decline attributable to these measures is much less than
indicated by the figures. Immunization and medical treatment
probably played only a secondary role in reducing airborne infectious disease deaths, with the two exceptions of diphtheria and
tuberculosis (McKeown, 1979, pp. 50-52). In the case of tuberculosis the majority of the reduction in mortality preceded the
introduction of streptomycin in 1948. However, it would be quite
inappropriate to omit recognition of the dramatically beneficial
effect this drug has had on fatality from tuberculous meningitis
and miliary tuberculosis.

The water- and food-borne diseases are the ones which are
likely to be reduced by prevention of exposure. The death rate

TABLE 4.4: Airborne diseases: fall in mortality since introduction of specific measures of prophylaxis or treatment: England and Wales

Causes	Total fall in standardized death rate between 1848–1854 and 1971	Fall by 1971 after introduction of specific measures	Fall by 1971 after introduction of specific measure as % of total fall
	a	b	$\frac{b}{a} \times 100$
Respiratory tuberculosis	2,888	409	14
Bronchitis, pneumonia, influenza	1,636	531	32
Whooping cough	422	43	10
Measles	342	50	15
Scarlet fever, diphtheria	1,016	307	30
Smallpox	263	263	100
Infections of ear, pharynx, larynx	73	65	89

From T. McKeown, *The Role of Medicine: Dream, Mirage or Nemesis?*, p. 51. Copyright © 1979 by Princeton University Press. Amended and reprinted by permission of Princeton University Press and Basil Blackwell, Ltd., Oxford, England.

from cholera, diarrhea, dysentery, nonrespiratory tuberculosis, typhoid, and typhus fell continuously from the second half of the 19th century. The one exception is gastroenteritis of infancy, which did not decline until the 20th century. There is no doubt that the fall in mortality from these diseases was due to the reduced exposure brought about by improvements in hygiene. These developments included purification of water, efficient disposal of sewage, and food hygiene. During the first half of the 19th century, the first two of these measures deteriorated due to population growth. Later in the century water and sewage systems were rebuilt. With airborne diseases, in contrast to water- and food-borne diseases, it is not possible to prevent exposure. Therefor, reduced exposure to infection could not have played an important part in the decline of airborne disease deaths (McKeown, 1979, pp. 56–57).

If the reduction in mortality from infectious diseases was not due to a change in their character, did not result from measures of immunization and therapy, and was affected little by reduced exposure before the latter part of the 19th century, then the remaining explanation is that improved health and nutrition modified the host's response to infections. There is no direct evidence to support this hypothesis; however, affirmative indirect evidence is persuasive. First is the relationship between malnutrition and infectious disease. It is well accepted that an adequate diet is the best protection against many infections. Second, the concurrent rapid growth in the population of many countries which differed in economic and other conditions suggests the possible operation of a common major change. The increase in food supplies resulting from advances in agriculture and transport in the 18th and 19th centuries was such a change. Most impressive is the fact that the large increase in the population of England and Wales was supported mainly on home-grown food, there being only a small import and export of food. The third proposition is that the increased food supply resulted in increased resistance to infection, thereby changing the host's susceptibility and reducing mortality from infectious diseases (McKeown, 1979, pp. 59–65).

The decline in noninfective conditions occurred after 1900, with the possible exceptions of infanticide and starvation. In the 20th century the reduction in mortality from noninfectious causes was considerable, but this has been concealed to some extent by the increases in death from lung cancer and myocardial infarction (McKeown, 1979, p. 66).

In the 20th century the heterogeneous class—prematurity, immaturity and other diseases of infancy—made the largest contribution to the fall in mortality from noninfectious conditions. This probably resulted from a number of factors, including a rising standard of living, improvement in maternal nutrition, better infant feeding and care, and improved obstetric care and management of the premature infant. This broad category of infant diseases contributed as much to the decline in infant mortality as did the infective condition, gastroenteritis. Next in magnitude were diseases classified as "other diseases," of which the largest reductions occurred in deaths due to alcoholism, rickets, and noninfective diseases of the respiratory system other than emphysema and asthma. These improvements are probably explained by less frequent drinking, improved nutrition, and better certification in the case of respiratory diseases. Treatment was responsible for reductions in some causes of death. Declines in "other diseases of the digestive system" were largely in those conditions now treated by surgery, such as gall bladder disease, intestinal obstruction, and hernia, and also with cirrhosis due to less alcohol consumption. The decline in deaths from violence, despite the increased incidence of accidents, is mainly attributable to surgery. The expla-

nation for the decline in noninfectious causes of death in the
20th century is more varied and less specific than for the infections.
Therapy played a major part in reducing deaths from some conditions (McKeown, 1979, pp. 66–68).

Prior to 1900 the decline in noninfectious causes of death was
probably due to reductions in infanticide and starvation. The
decline in infanticide, although poorly documented, probably occurred during the 19th century. It was associated with the growth
in foundling hospitals and asylums for exposed and deserted young
children. The major reason for the decline was the growth of
contraceptive practices, which reduced the number of unwanted
births (McKeown, 1979, pp. 68–70).

Determinants of Health

McKeown's historical analysis provides a general introduction to
the determinants of health and the risk of disease. Contrary to
much popular thought, medical measures probably have played a
relatively small part in the changing pattern of mortality and life
expectancy. The major contribution to the decline in mortality
from infectious disease has been environmental. Increased food
production in the 18th and 19th centuries led to improved nutrition and reduced susceptibility to infectious disease. Initial agricultural developments late in the 17th century, such as the
introduction of new crops and more effective application of traditional farming methods, led to increased production. Scientific
advances, such as mechanization and chemical fertilizers, brought
by the industrial revolution, added to the agricultural growth
during the second half of the 19th century. These agricultural
developments were not designed for health purposes, whereas the
improvements introduced by the sanitary reformers in the 1870s
were expressly for purposes of hygiene. The principal sanitary
changes were purification of water and sewage disposal. Food
hygiene was greatly improved after 1900. Most important was the
better quality of milk effected through sterilization, bottling, and
safe transport. During the 18th and 19th centuries other environmental changes were taking place; industries were developing
and the rural landscape was becoming urbanized. Interestingly,
the adverse health effects of these developments were offset by
the factors which caused the decline in mortality. The second
major determinant of improved health was behavioral. Altered
reproductive behavior, which was not introduced for health pur-

poses, led to a decline in the birth rate. If this had not occurred the population of Britain today would be 140 million rather than 50 million. Limitation of birth was the essential component without which the benefits of the increased food production would have been negated. In addition, the restraint on reproduction probably affected infanticide directly. In summary, therefore, the determinants of the modern transformation of health over the past three centuries were improvements in nutrition since about 1700, hygienic measures since late in the 19th century, vaccination and therapy in the 20th century, and change in reproductive behavior. When advances in nutrition and hygiene are grouped together as environmental factors the influences responsible for the fall in mortality and the increase in life expectancy were environmental, behavioral, and therapeutic. They were introduced in the 18th, 19th, and 20th centuries, respectively. Their order of introduction is also that of their effectiveness (McKeown, 1979, pp. 74-78).

RISK AND NATURAL HISTORY

The determinants of health are one aspect of health. They are one component in interactions between people and their environment. Although a determinant such as poor nutrition, for example, can cause disease, this does not result in all cases. A given diet may cause disease in one individual while its effect in a second may be undetectable. If such effects were uniform the relationship between determinants and the host would have no unknowns. The variation in the occurrence of disease, due to potentially harmful factors, necessitates understanding both the risk relationships between these factors and the host population, as well as the subsequent course of disease.

Definitions

The concept of risk is based on the existence of an association between disease and some attribute or risk factor. In a group of people who all share the same risk factor, the incidence of disease is greater than would occur in the absence of the risk factor. Although a larger proportion of the group than expected develop the disease, there are many who remain disease-free. A common example of this is the occurrence of lung cancer among smokers. Along with cases of lung cancer are many smokers who never develop the disease. Risk only implies association and not causation. This is not to say that some risk factors, for example, irradiation, asbestos, or cigarettes, are not causative agents. A risk factor, in contrast to the cause of a disease, does not explain why the disease has developed, or why some individuals exposed to the risk factor do not become ill. Basic to the concept of risk is a temporal relationship in which the presence of the risk factor precedes development of disease. That is, there is an early stage in the natural history of disease when the only distinction which can be made between individuals is their susceptibility in terms of the presence or absence of risk factors. The sequence of steps that results in the individuals who develop disease constitute the natural history of disease.

The natural history of disease can be defined as "the time course of the interaction between man, causal factors, and the rest of the environment, beginning with the biologic onset of the disease and ending with the outcomes of recovery, death or some other state of physical, social or emotional function" (Department of Clinical Epidemiology, 1981a, pp. 869–870). It is useful to distinguish five stages within this time course. The first is the stage of susceptibility, when a proportion of individuals at increased risk to disease can be identified. This is followed by the stage of earliest pathological change at which time diagnosis is not usually possible. In the third stage the patient is asymptomatic; early diagnosis is possible through screening or diagnostic testing. The fourth is the usual time of diagnosis, at which stage symptoms appear and the patient seeks clinical help. In the final stage, the outcomes of the disease manifest themselves. The patient may die, recover, or suffer from some chronic disease state (Hutchinson, 1960).

The most important clinical application of the natural history concerns prognosis. The prognosis of disease describes the likelihood of various disease outcomes occurring in terms of characteristics of the clinical course. The importance of temporality to the concept of risk also applies to prognosis.

While this general scheme applies to both chronic and infectious diseases, there are some differences between the two types of disease. The cause of infectious disease is usually one specific organism, whereas a number of risk factors are frequently associated with chronic diseases and the cause is commonly unknown. With infectious disease, in contrast to chronic disorders, the interval between exposure to the cause and clinical illness is known, the outcome can be predicted accurately, and a recurrence is often prevented through acquired immunity.

Methods

The methodological aspects of risk, causation, and prognosis stem from the need to understand associations between health outcomes and predisposing factors. The question is whether or not an observed association is causal. When two observations are found to be associated, there are four possible explanations for this. For purposes of illustration, assume the two factors to be A and B. The four possible relationships between A and B are:

A causes B
B causes A
C causes B
The association is an artefact

In the first case A causes B. Alternatively, a causal relationship may exist but the direction is reversed so that B causes A. The third possibility is that a third factor, C, or confounding variable, is responsible. In this case C causes B as well as being associated with A. This results in A being associated with B, but without the relationship being causal. Interference from confounding variables is commonly caused by various types of bias which the researcher fails to control. The fourth explanation is that the association is due to a methodological error and is therefore artefactual. When presented with an association between two factors A and B the question of whether A is responsible for B can be answered with confidence only when the other possible explanations have been shown to be quite improbable. Commonly the inappropriate claim is made that one factor causes another when this cannot be substantiated in terms of rejecting the other possible explanations. For this reason it is particularly important to have criteria to assist in assessing whether an observed association can be accepted as being causal. It is relevant to recognize that causation in medicine is often very difficult to prove.

In the case of chronic disease, the existence of multiple risk factors and the absence of a single causative agent has made the identification of etiological factors particularly difficult. On the other hand, the bacterial causation of infectious disease is one aspect of medicine in which causation has been identified with a high degree of confidence. The scientific approach to bacterial causation was established by Robert Koch (Volk & Wheeler, 1984).

In the late 19th century Koch's postulates provided specific criteria for evaluating evidence concerning identification of the bacterial cause of infectious disease. A more general set of criteria was first defined by Sir Austin Bradford Hill (Hill, 1977, pp. 285–296) to provide a methodological framework for assessing evidence for causation. These criteria follow:

1. *Is there evidence from true experiments in humans?* The first and singularly most important criterion is evidence from a randomized trial. This type of study is designed to control all the possible reasons for two variables, A and B, being associated with the obvious exception of the relationship under investigation, namely that A causes B. The first step in this type of research design is the identification of a homogeneous group in which no members have the outcome of interest. Half the group is then allocated randomly to be exposed to the "causative" factor under investigation. The whole group is followed for a period of time and examined for the occurrence of the outcome. The incidence rate of the outcome in the exposed subgroup is compared with that in the unexposed subgroup. The basic structure of this analysis is that of a 2 × 2 table as shown in Figure 4.3. The design of the randomized trial is summarized in Figure 4.4.

When a true experiment has not been carried out, it is important to consider the type of research designs that have been employed. Research designs vary in strength. The basic types of design, in order of decreasing strength, are the cohort analytic study, case-control, analytic survey, and nonanalytic survey or case series. The

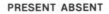

OUTCOME

PRESENT ABSENT

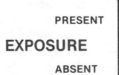

PRESENT | a   b

EXPOSURE

ABSENT | c   d

FIGURE 4–3 The two by two table.

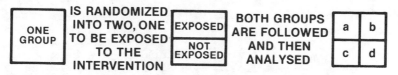

FIGURE 4–4 Basic design of a randomized trial.

cohort study is shown in Figure 4.5. It is similar to the experiment in that the subjects are followed over a period of time. However, its weakness is the potential for the two groups (the exposed and the unexposed) to be dissimilar in some important way in addition to the presence of the exposure. This can occur because the basis on which the group is subdivided into an exposed and unexposed subgroup is unknown and has not been done randomly. In the case-control design, shown in Figure 4.6, the two study groups are selected in terms of the presence of the outcome. A group of cases with the outcome of interest is compared with one or more comparison groups which do not have the outcome. This design is open to a number of sources of bias (Sackett, 1979). In the analytic survey one group of individuals is examined in terms of the presence or absence of exposure and outcome. In addition to important bias problems, it can lack statistical power due to very small numbers in some cells of the 2×2 table. (See Figure 4.7.) Finally, the case series or nonanalytic survey is useful for generating questions and hypotheses, but as it lacks a comparison group it cannot be used for hypothesis testing. (See Figure 4.8.) In summary, the greatest reliance can be placed on the randomized trial, but as experimental evidence is frequently unavailable cautious use often needs to be made of data from studies with less strength and greater possibility of bias.

2. *Is the association strong?* Strength here refers to the likelihood of the outcome being greater for individuals with the exposure of interest than among individuals in whom the exposure is absent. The higher the likelihood, the greater the strength.

There are different methods for calculating the strength of an association. In a randomized trial and a cohort study, strength can

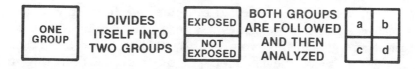

FIGURE 4–5 Basic design of a cohort study.

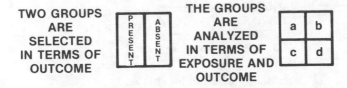

FIGURE 4–6 Basic design of a case-control study.

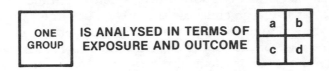

FIGURE 4–7 Basic design of an analytic survey.

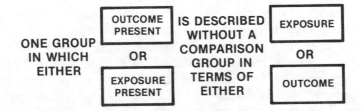

FIGURE 4–8 Basic design of a nonanalytic survey or case-series.

be calculated directly by means of comparing outcome rates in exposed and unexposed persons using the relative risks formula:

$$\left(\frac{a}{a+b}\right)\bigg/\left(\frac{c}{c+d}\right)$$

In case-control studies and analytic surveys the relative odds formula, ad/bc, should be used rather than relative risk. These studies, in contrast to a randomized trial or cohort study, do not measure incidence, and it is therefore inappropriate to employ a formula constructed from incidence rates such as relative risk. A relative odds or relative risk of 1 indicates there is no association. A positive association is reflected by figures greater than one, and a negative association by figures less than one. Strength increases as the figure gets further from one. A relative risk of 2 indicates that there is twice the likelihood of the outcome occurring in the presence of the exposure of interest.

3. *Is the association consistent from study to study?* The repeated demonstration of an association between the exposure and outcome from study to study using different methods, different subjects in different places, and at different times all indicate consistency.

4. *Is the temporal relationship correct?* When contact with the exposure of interest precedes development of the outcome the temporal relationship is correct. Only randomized trials and cohort studies are capable of assuring that the temporal relationship is appropriate.

5. *Is there a dose-response gradient?* For this criterion to be met it is necessary to demonstrate an increase in the strength of association between exposure and outcome with an increase in the quantity of exposure. Only studies which evaluate at least two levels of exposure are capable of demonstrating a gradient.

6. *Does the association make epidemiologic sense?* This criterion is met when the association is consistent with current understanding of the determinants and distribution of disease in terms of person, place, and time.

7. *Does the association make biologic sense?* Is the association consistent with current understanding of the response of cells, tissues, organs, and organisms to stimuli?

8. *Is the association specific?* This criterion is met when the observed association is limited to a specific exposure and a specific outcome.

9. *Analogy.* Is the association analogous to a previously proven causal association?

While these criteria are not of equal importance each one reflects a dimension to the extensive scientific argument needed before a relationship is accepted as causal. Following experimental evidence the criteria concerning the strength of association, consistency, temporality, and a dose-response gradient are the most important (Department of Clinical Epidemiology, 1981b). The other criteria are of lesser value.

In addition to causation, assessment of the prognosis of existing disease is of major importance to the clinician. Most of the inconsistencies in the investigation of the clinical course of illness arise from how patients are selected for study and followed up. Similar to the above causation guidelines, the following set of methodological criteria for assessing studies of prognosis provides a standard by which to judge evidence concerning the probability of various outcomes developing in patients with diagnosed disease (Department of Clinical Epidemiology, 1981a).

1. *Was an inception cohort assembled?* In studies of prognosis all the patients in the study should be entered at an early and uniform point in the clinical course of the disease. Such a group is an inception cohort. This type of selection aims at minimizing exclusion from the study those patients who either succumb or completely recover early in the clinical course. Inception cohorts can be defined at times such as when the first unambiguous symptoms are present or when therapy is started. Failure to assemble an inception cohort can lead to results indicating either a more pessimistic outlook or a prognosis more favorable than actually exists.

2. *Was the referral pattern described?* In order to make appropriate use of a study it is necessary to be able to identify whether the results apply to patients in your own practice. For this reason it is important that the source and pattern of referral of patients be described. For example, tertiary centers attract serious and rare cases compared with primary care units, where the distribution of patients reflects more closely the pattern of disease in the general community. Studies of prognosis in these two settings would not be comparable. The method of selecting patients for studies of prognosis can lead to several types of bias of which the clinician should be aware (Sackett, 1979; Sackett and Whelan, 1980).

3. *Was complete follow-up achieved?* All patients should be accounted for at the end of a study and their clinical outcome known. Reasons for patients being lost from a study can often relate to important clinical events such as death, recovery, or a change in therapy. The loss of such patients can seriously distort the results.

4. *Were objective outcome criteria developed and used?* Because clinical disagreement is common (Department of Clinical Epidemiology, 1980a) it is necessary to assure that the reported clinical outcomes are accurate. The minimum requirements for this are the description of explicit outcome criteria plus their consistent application.

5. *Was the outcome assessment "blind"?* The investigators assessing patient outcomes should be "blind" to the other features of the patient. For example, awareness of a presumably important prognostic factor can lead to more frequent or detailed clinical

examination; judgement in assessing diagnostic specimens can be affected by knowledge of the clinical history.

6. *Was adjustment for extraneous prognostic factors carried out?* This criterion refers to the presence of confounding variables mentioned earlier in this section. It is important to exclude the possibility that a factor other than a significant clinical characteristic has led to the observed patient outcome.

The criteria for studies of prognosis and those concerning causation identify the major research prerequisites for evidence pertaining to these two aspects of the natural history of disease. The methodological aspects of risk are particularly important given the multiple sources of error and bias in research into etiology and prognosis.

SUMMARY

This chapter has provided a historical and methodological introduction to the determinants of health. From the historical perspective a wide range of factors have contributed over recent centuries to a dramatic increase in life expectancy and decline in mortality. Prior to this century environmental and behavioral factors exerted the principal influence on the decline in infectious diseases. During this century the role of immunization and therapy has contributed to declines in both infectious and chronic disease. Reference has also been made to the deleterious effect of certain human behavior which has played a part in the epidemic increases in deaths from myocardial infarction and lung cancer. Overall, the role of scientific medicine in promoting health is less than is commonly assumed.

In the next chapters the focus will be on current causes of disease and ill health. As a preamble to this the methodological difficulties encountered in evaluating evidence of causation and prognosis have been discussed. While the interpretations of much published research are inadequately substantiated, the reader of scientific literature can guard against this by making his or her own interpretations through the use of methodological criteria. Against this general background of awareness of the multifactorial etiology of much disease and an attitude of methodological skepticism, some specific causes of current diseases will be examined.

Chapter 5

Risks II: Causes of Disease

Disease develops from the effect of factors which are both internal and external to the human host. The interaction between these factors has been shown to be of particular importance in determining the occurrence of infectious disease. In this chapter the focus is on the causes of current diseases which are largely noninfectious but for which the relationship between the host and causative agents is also very important. Three categories of cause of disease will be described: heredity and constitutional factors; behavior and life style; and environmental factors which are mainly outside the control of the individual. The purpose is to describe the major causes of disease within these three categories and to consider the nature of the underlying evidence.

HEREDITARY FACTORS

Diseases can occur in two ways. Either they are determined genetically or, despite normal genes, there is an inability to adapt to the environment. Genetic diseases are determined at the time of fertilization, whereas environmental disorders develop any time thereafter, either prenatally or during postnatal life.

Among the genetic disorders three categories can be identified. First there are single-gene disorders, which are inherited according to Mendelian principles as dominant, recessive, or x-linked diseases. They include conditions such as Turner's and Kleinfelter's syndromes, hemophilia, phenylketonuria, sickle cell disease, and fibrocystic disease. When fertility is low or absent, the number of these conditions in the population is reduced by natural selection. The continued presence of diseases such as hemophilia is due to new mutations. The second group comprises those disorders due to chromosomal aberrations, and which can be identified under the microscope. It is estimated that they are present in 5% of embryos at the beginning of pregnancy, but due to the majority being lost through abortion, few occur among live births. The commonest chromosomal disorder is Down's syndrome. The overall incidence of diseases due to single-gene disorders and chromosomal aberrations is approximately 0.5% of live births. The third category of hereditary disease is an ill-defined and poorly understood group. It comprises the majority of diseases determined at fertilization, the occurrence of which can only be inferred. McKeown reasons that if the maximum duration of life is genetically programmed, and is therefore determined at fertilization, it is reasonable to assume that some diseases and disabilities associated with the end of life are similarly determined. If this proposition is accepted, then much of the organ degeneration and failure associated with old age would be attributed to multiple genes programmed at fertilization. This could include breakdown of nonessential organs such as eyes, ears, or joints, or the partial failures of essential organs such as brain, heart, or kidneys, usually due to vascular degeneration (McKeown, 1979, pp. 14-15).

In addition to this potentially genetic component of chronic disease, it is well established that most congenital malformations and the common physical and mental diseases result from exposure to environmental factors (McKeown, 1979, p. 79).

Although environmental exposure causes disease in many individuals, it does not have this effect on everyone who is exposed, indicating variability in individual susceptibility to environmental factors.

The majority of diseases are multifactorial in etiology and result from an interaction of multiple genetic and environmental factors. Identification of the respective contribution of heredity and environment to disease is particularly difficult. This requires the effect of one of the two sets of factors to be controlled while the effect of the other is evaluated. Such an approach is rendered impossible, or at least very difficult, when environmental factors are multiple and genetic factors cannot be identified directly (McKeown, 1979, pp. 16-20). Despite these constraints there is a growing body of knowledge concerning the role of specific environmental factors in the cause of disease. Much of this research is conducted on populations which are heterogeneous in terms of genetic susceptibility.

BEHAVIOR AND LIFE STYLE

The environmental factors to which people are exposed are complex and varied. These factors generally fall into one of two broad categories. Behavior and life style refer to environmental factors which are usually under the control of the individual. Exposure to the other environmental factors is generally beyond individual choice. This second group will be described in the next section. — Behavior and life style are those activities, habits, and customs which characterize an individual's everyday life. Activities such as smoking, drinking, eating, driving, and social and recreational activities are all of particular relevance to health because they affect the individual's environment. Selected aspects of life style will be considered.

Smoking

The harmful effects of smoking were not given general attention until 1950. In that year three reports identified an increased incidence of lung cancer in smokers (Doll & Hill, 1950; Levin, Goldstein, & Gerhardt, 1950; Wynder & Graham, 1950). While clinical suspicion of the deleterious effect of cigarettes dates back to at least the early 1900's, this was not adequately documented until after World War II. Since then the number and efficiency of studies have proliferated such that the current state of knowledge rests on highly consistent findings from many case-control studies and a number of cohort studies.

In the U.S. Veterans Study (Rogot & Murray, 1980) nearly 300,000 individuals holding U.S. government life insurance policies in December 1953 were followed for 16 years. The association between smoking and causes of death was analyzed. Mortality ratios for current smokers compared with nonsmokers, summarized in Table 5.1, were greater than 1.0 for nearly all causes of death. The highest mortality ratios were 14.82 for emphysema, 14.05 for cancer of the pharynx, 11.49 for cancer of the lung and bronchus, 6.43 for cancer of the esophagus, 5.57 for cor pulmonale, 5.23 for aortic aneurysm, and 5.11 for bronchitis. For all causes of death the mortality ratio was 1.73. Although the mortality ratio for cardiovascular disease was less than this, more than 50% (nearly 8,000 deaths) of all 15,286 excess deaths due to current smoking were from cardiovascular disease. Approximately 5,000 of these were from coronary heart disease. Of all excess deaths from current smoking the proportions from other major diseases were 26% from all cancers, 16% from lung cancer, 11% from all respiratory diseases, and 8% from bronchitis and emphysema.

The death rate from the majority of causes increases with the amount of tobacco smoked. This positive gradient exists for both current and ex-smokers. The age-specific death rates from ischemic heart disease in the British Doctors' 20-year follow-up study (Doll & Peto, 1976) demonstrate this clearly (see Table 5.2). The gradient is quite evident for each age group up to age 64. There is also a negative gradient demonstrated by the decline in deaths among ex-smokers; this progresses with the years since smoking stopped. In Table 5.3 the number of deaths among ex-smokers is shown as a percentage of the number of expected deaths in continuing smokers according to years since ceasing to smoke. This inverse relationship exists for all causes of death among those aged under 65 as well as those older than 65. Possible exceptions to this are deaths from aortic aneurysm, bronchitis, emphysema, and lung cancer (Rogot & Murray, 1980).

The role of smoking as a cause of disease is now well established. Cigarettes are undoubtedly one of the leading known causes of sickness in this century. The effects of smoke inhaled passively from the cigarettes of others also leads to increased death rates (Hirayama, 1981). This finding, combined with the socioeconomic burden on society of smoking-induced disease, presents a major ethical problem associated with smoking.

TABLE 5.1: Mortality Ratios Among Current Smokers for Selected Causes of Death, U.S. Veterans Study 1954–1969

Causes of Death	Mortality Ratios for Current Smokers
All causes	1.73
Cardiovascular diseases	1.58
Cancers, all sites	2.12
Coronary heart disease	1.58
Stroke	1.32
Influenza and pneumonia	1.78
Aortic aneurysm	5.23
Parkinson's disease	0.32
Bronchitis and emphysema	12.07
Lung cancer	11.28

From E. Rogot and J.L. Murray, 1980. Smoking and causes of death among U.S. veterans: 16 years of observation. *Public Health Reports* 95(3):221. Reproduced by permission from *Public Health Reports*.

TABLE 5.2: Age-specific annual death rates from ischemic heart disease by number of cigarettes smoked, male British doctors

Age (in years)	Non smokers	Annual Death Rate per 100,000 Men* Current Smokers, Smoking Only Cigarettes (no. per day)		
		1–14	15–24	≥25
<45	7	46	61	104
45 – 54	118	220	368	393
55 – 64	531	742	819	1025
65 – 74	1190	1866	1511	1731
75 +	2432	2719	2466	3247

* Indirectly standardized for age to make the four entries in any one line comparable.
From R. Doll and R. Peto, 1976. Mortality in relation to smoking: 20 years' observations on male British doctors. *British Medical Journal* 2: 1529. Reproduced by permission from the *British Medical Journal* and the authors.

TABLE 5.3: Mortality in ex-cigarette smokers compared with mortality in continuing cigarette smokers, male British doctors

Cause of Death	No. of Deaths as % of No. Expected in Continuing Cigarette Smokers Years Since Smoking Stopped			
	<5	5 – 9	10 – 14	≥15
All causes at 30 – 64 years	86	80	69	56
All causes at 65 and over	87	89	78	71

Source: Data from Doll and Peto 1976, p. 1531.

Despite the extensive justification for not smoking the consumption of tobacco per adult is continuing to increase around the world. The United States has the highest per capita consumption of tobacco, followed by Canada (World Health Organization, 1979, pp. 92–93). This trend differs for males and females. Since 1961, tobacco consumption for Canadian males has been steady, but for females it increased up to 1975. In comparison, some favorable trends in the proportion of the population who smoke are beginning to appear. Since 1965 the proportion of smokers in Canada has been declining due to fewer males smoking. The proportion of female smokers has remained steady except for an increasing proportion of females 15 to 19 years who smoke. Canadians with the highest smoking rate are those aged between 20 and 24 years and alcohol drinkers of all ages. The elderly have the lowest rate of smoking (Ableson, Paddon, & Strohmenger, 1983, p. 30; Statistics Canada, 1981b, Tables 11 and 22).

Alcohol

Alcohol consumption is thought to play a role in approximately 10% of all deaths in Canada. In 1978 there were 2,520 deaths caused directly by alcohol. In 5,668 violent deaths alcohol was an associated factor, and there is evidence that alcohol may have played a role in 10,142 other deaths (Ableson, Paddon, & Strohmenger, 1983, p. 23). In addition to alcohol consumption being associated with increased mortality there is growing evidence that a moderate intake may be beneficial to health. One such study of British male civil servants found the mortality rate to be lower in moderate drinkers than in either nondrinkers or individuals drinking over 34 grams of alcohol per day (Marmot et al., 1981). The relative risk of death for alcohol consumption shown in Table 5.4 indicates a higher cardiovascular mortality among nondrinkers and an excess of noncardiovascular deaths among heavy drinkers.

Within the general impact of mortality are a number of specific health effects of alcohol. There is a well-documented relationship between a country's per capita alcohol consumption and both mortality and morbidity. Deaths from cirrhosis, hospital admissions due to alcoholism and alcoholic psychosis, and convictions for various forms of unlawful behavior are all positively associated with national alcohol consumption (Smith, 1981b). The contribution of alcohol to accidents is particularly notable. Table 5.5 shows figures indicating that alcohol was associated with approx-

TABLE 5.4: Relative risk of death according to alcohol consumption adjusting for age, smoking habit, diastolic blood pressure, plasma cholesterol concentration, and grade of employment, British male civil servants

Cause of Death	Alcohol Consumption (g/day)			
	0	0.1–9	9.1–34	>34
Cardiovascular	2.1	1.0	1.5	0.9
Non-cardiovascular	1.0	1.0	0.5	2.1
Total*	1.6	1.0	1.0	1.5

* Fitting a quadratic (U-shaped) curve to these relative risks yields $x_1^2 = 3.41$ (p = 0.065) and the overall test between alcohol categories yields $x_1^2 = 3.75$, i.e., the quadratic relationship accounts for most of the differences between categories.

From M.G. Marmot, G. Rose, M.J. Shipley, & B.J. Thomas, 1981. Alcohol and mortality: A U-shaped curve. *Lancet* 1(8220, Pt. 1):582. Reproduced by permission from The Lancet Ltd.

imately one third of fatal motor vehicle accidents in Ontario in
1980 and 1981. Fatalities among drivers involve alcohol consumption in more than 50% of cases (Ministry of Transportation,
1981).

In contrast, cancer incidence is affected only to a small extent
by alcohol alone. However, alcohol combined with smoking seems
to multiply the carcinogenic effect of tobacco smoke on the mouth,
pharynx, larynx, and esophagus. In the case of esophageal cancer,
the relative risk for heavy smokers is approximately 6, and when
combined with heavy alcohol consumption this risk increases to
over 44 (Tuyns, Pequignot, & Jensen 1977). Cancers of the four
above-mentioned sites related to alcohol consumption account for
7% of all cancer deaths in males and 3% in women. Of all cancer
deaths, approximately 3% can be attributed to alcohol (Doll &
Peto, 1981, p. 1225).

In addition to the objective and measurable health effects of
alcohol there are many emotional and social problems associated
with excessive drinking (Health and Welfare Canada, 1976). In
terms of reducing the quality of life alcohol is a major factor.

Over the past 30 years the consumption of alcohol has increased
very considerably in North America and in much of Europe. Per
capita consumption has at least doubled in several countries, such
as Canada, West Germany, and The Netherlands; however, since
1975 this increase has become less noticeable (Ableson, Paddon,
& Strohmenger, 1983, pp. 23–24).

TABLE 5.5: Alcohol consumption of drivers in motor vehicle accidents, Ontario, 1980 and 1981

Condition of Driver	Type of Motor Vehicle Accident		
	All Accidents %	Fatal Accidents %	Driver Fatalities* %
Apparently normal	83	56	44
Impaired by alcohol	3	18	42
Had been drinking	6	13	14
Other or unknown	8	13	—
Total	100	100	100

* Excludes cases where data on alcohol consumption were not provided.
Source: Ministry of Transportation and Communications, 1981, p. 14.

In summary, alcohol is an important contributor to ill health, disease, and disability. For this reason, and because its use is prevalent, the relevance of alcohol is both real and current.

Diet

The investigation of the health effects of diet is more complex than for smoking or alcohol. While only a proportion of society smokes or drinks, eating is ubiquitous and is necessary in order to sustain life. The variability in the quantity and composition of diet among populations and individuals is great, and the health effects of diet relate to both deficiencies and excesses of food, as well as to its composition.

A lack of food leads to starvation. The failure of crops such as that preceding the Irish Potato Famine, the deliberate destruction of farms and fields in war, and the prescribed starvation of concentration camps are florid examples of the need for food.

Lesser degrees of dietary insufficiency have a variety of effects. Deficiency of specific dietary components produces well-recognized disease states such as scurvy, rickets, beri-beri, pellagra, kwashiorkor, and marasmus. A general state of undernutrition increases an individual's susceptibility to infectious disease. Malnutrition is thought to be one of the major factors underlying the high mortality from infectious disease which controlled world population prior to the modern rise in population (McKeown, 1976, pp. 128-142). Diet also has an important effect at the level of growth and development. In an experiment conducted in 1926, schoolchildren who were considered to be taking an inadequate diet were found to have a significant increase in height and weight when given food supplements (Mann, 1926). Consistent with this, in Britain today children and adolescents are taller and heavier than they were at the turn of the century. Since that time the average diet has improved (McKeown & Lowe, 1966, pp. 123-126).

During this century the role of diet in health has taken on an added dimension. Generally, the dietary insufficiencies of the past have been replaced by overeating and health problems associated with affluence. In a prospective study of behavior and health Belloc and Breslow (1972) observed that the following seven behaviors were associated with health and longevity: (1) not smoking cigarettes, (2) sleeping 7 hours a day, (3) eating breakfast, (4) keeping weight down, (5) drinking moderately, (6) exercising daily, and (7) not eating between meals. It is interesting to note that three of the seven behaviors, not including alcohol consumption, concern diet. One specific consequence of dietary excess is obesity. Based on life insurance statistics, there is twice the mortality rate among individuals 25% heavier than the average for their age and sex (McKeown & Lowe, 1966, p. 122). In addition to mortality and obesity the incidence of a large number of diseases is thought to be influenced by a modern western diet. Among these diseases are ischemic heart disease, diabetes mellitus, and cancer. Accidents are higher among the obese, probably because of reduced agility. It is estimated that 35% of cancer deaths are due to dietary factors (Doll & Peto, 1981, p. 1256). Burkitt (1969), based on comparisons of Africa with Western countries, proposes that a low fiber diet is responsible for diseases such as appendicitis, diverticular disease, adenomatous polyps of the bowel and colon, and rectal cancer. The role of diet in some of the major diseases will be discussed in more depth in the next chapter.

There is little question that diet is a major factor in health. However, there is much uncertainty about the exact nature of this effect, including the relationship of diet with other causative factors.

Exercise

Exercise is one form of behavior in this series of life style activities which is both pleasurable and healthy. The question deserving an answer is, to what degree does exercise promote health? Undoubtedly exercise brings direct benefits in the form of a sense of well-being in addition to promoting social contact and relaxation.

In terms of disease prevention, research has focused principally on exercise as a protection against ischemic heart disease. Physiologically, such an association is reasonable. The original investigation on the subject was conducted by Morris et al. (1953). They studied prospectively 31,000 employees of the London Transport Executive and observed an association between physical activity at work and protection against fatal heart attacks. Subsequently it was shown that the relative risk of developing coronary disease among men performing vigorous leisure-time exercise was about one third that in comparable men who did not perform such exercise. This benefit was not shown for moderate exercise (Morris et al., 1973). In one of a number of studies with comparable findings the relative risk of heart attack for males with an energy expenditure below 2,000 kilocalories per week was 1.64 compared with those with an energy expenditure above this level. The relative risk for nonfatal heart attacks among the lower energy expenditure group compared with those with a higher expenditure was 1.48, and for fatal heart attacks the relative risk was 2.01. Exercise was independent of other risk factors such as smoking and hypertension (Paffenbarger, Wing, & Hyde, 1978).

In summary, the performance of physical exercise benefits both the quality of life and the incidence of coronary heart disease; however, the latter depends upon an adequate level of energy expenditure.

Reproductive and Sexual Behavior

The indirect effect of reduced family size on the modern decline in mortality has already been described. In terms of the direct influence of reproductive and sexual behavior on disease, an association has been observed with several female cancers, including cancer of the cervix, breast, endometrium, and ovary. The risk of cancer of the cervix is increased by both early intercourse and increasing numbers of sexual partners (Rokin, 1981). Cancer of the ovary, endometrium, and breast are all somewhat less common in women who have borne children early than in women who have had no children (Doll & Peto, 1981, p. 1237). Cancer of the breast in parous women becomes progressively less likely as the age of first pregnancy decreases (MacMahon, Cole, & Brown, 1973).

Driving Behavior

A large proportion of motor vehicle accidents are considered to be the result of human behavior. Major factors in the occurrence and severity of traffic accidents include drinking and driving (Ministry of Transportation, 1981) and failure to use seat belts (Anderson, 1967). Despite these facts, the prevalence of these behaviors remains high. Over 30% of drivers in all fatal car accidents in Ontario in 1981 had been drinking alcohol (Ministry of Transportation, 1981), and in 1977 it was estimated that less than 30% of Canadians wore seat belts while driving (Ableson, Paddon, & Strohmenger, 1983, p. 45).

Social Relationships

The final aspect of life style to be considered is the individual's social network. It is important to recognize that social relationships may depend upon factors beyond individual volition. It may be an oversimplification to consider them as a form of behavioral risk factor comparable to smoking or eating, for example. Acknowledging this uncertainty, it is relevant to consider in this section the documented association between social networks and health. Mortality rates have been found to increase as social ties decrease (Blazer, 1982; Berkman & Syme, 1979). In a 9-year prospective study death rates in males with the fewest social relationships were more than twice as high as among individuals with an extensive social network. For females the death rate was nearly three times higher in the socially isolated (Berkman & Syme, 1979). (See Table 2.4.) The role of social networks is not limited to the probable effect on mortality. It can be argued that communication and interaction among people is fundamental to human existence, without which life loses its value, and as quality of life receives more consideration as an important dimension to health we will need to expand our knowledge of the social aspects of health. This will require investigation into such questions as the role of social relationships in health, the factors influencing social networks, and the effects other aspects of lifestyle have upon social interaction. Activities such as smoking, drinking, eating, exercising, sexual relations, and driving cars all involve social behavior.

Discussion

In summary, there is much evidence relating life style to disease and disability. Heart disease is affected by smoking, diet, and exercise; cancer is affected by smoking, diet, sexual and reproductive behavior, and alcohol; and the rate and severity of accidents are strongly influenced by alcohol consumption and seat belt usage. To a large degree these behaviors are controlled by the individual; however, not all diseases are closely related to life style.

ENVIRONMENTAL FACTORS

For the purposes of considering environmental health effects other than life style the environment can be subdivided into three parts.

The first, about which the most is known, is the work environment. The second is the home and neighborhood environment, the health effects of which are little understood. The third is pollution of all aspects of the environment from both public and private sources.

Industrial growth, urbanization, and technological advances have made the modern environment extremely complex from many points of view, not least of which is the relationship of environment to health. Detailed consideration of this is well beyond the purpose of this document. However, this section aims to identify the overall role in health played by environmental factors.

Occupational Environment

Frank occupational disease is less common today than in the early part of this century (McKeown & Lowe, 1966, p. 84). The numerous forms of poisoning, pneumoconiosis, and occupational skin diseases, among others, are much less prevalent than previously. Today the major occupational health problems are the occurrence of physical disability due to injury and the actual and potential problem of occupational carcinogens.

Cancer due to work place exposure is both an old and a new problem. In 1775 Percivall Pott (1775) published his observations of scrotal cancer in chimney sweeps. By World War I occupational cancer of skin, bronchus, bladder, palate, lip, and buccal cavity had been recognized (Doll, 1980). Such observations and the search for occupational hazards in general have been the major source of knowledge of causes of human cancer (Doll & Peto, 1981, p. 1238). The occupational substances which have been shown to be carcinogenic are listed in Table 5.6. Each of these substances produces a specific cancer rather than having a general effect on malignancy. In addition to these known carcinogens, there are many new substances, mostly synthetic chemicals, which have been produced at a rapidly increasing rate since World War II (Davis & Magee, 1979). These substances are inadequately understood in terms of their toxicity. A major reason for a lack of knowledge of their carcinogenicity is the delay of at least 20 years between exposure to a carcinogen and the development of many cancers. This fact, combined with the disappearance of some occupations, the introduction of others, the production of many new potential carcinogens, and increased automation in industry, all make it impossible, without special data gathering, to make a

precise estimate of the proportion of cancers attributable to occupation (Doll & Peto, 1981, p. 1239).

Doll and Peto point out that nationally representative studies
of cancer, including thorough occupational histories, are needed
in order to understand the role of occupation in cancer. They
propose that until such case-control studies are in place, an estimate
can be made through considering each type of cancer separately

TABLE 5.6: Established Occupational Causes of Cancer

Agent	Site of Cancer	Occupation
Aromatic amines	Bladder	Dye manufacturers, rubber workers, coal gas manufacturers
Arsenic*	Skin, lung	Copper and cobalt smelters, arsenical pesticide manufacturers, some gold miners
Asbestos	Lung, pleura, peritoneum	Asbestos miners, asbestos textile manufacturers, asbestos insulation workers, certain shipyard workers
Benzene	Marrow	Workers with glues and varnishes
Bischloromethyl ether	Lung	Makers of ion-exchange resins
Cadmium*	Prostate	Cadmium workers
Chromium*	Lung	Manufacturers of chromates from chrome ore, pigment manufacturers
Ionizing radia-tions	Lung	Uranium and some other miners
	Bone	Luminizers
	Marrow, all sites	Radiologists, radiographers
Isopropyl oil	Nasal sinuses	Isopropyl alcohol manufacturers
Mustard gas	Larynx, lung	Poison gas manufacturers
Nickel*	Nasal sinuses, lung	Nickel refiners
Polycyclic hydrocarbons in soot, tar, oil	Skin, scrotum, lung	Coal gas manufacturers, roofers, asphalters, aluminum refiners, many groups selectively exposed to certain tars and oils
UV light	Skin	Farmers, seamen
Vinyl chloride	Liver	PVC manufacturers
**	Nasal sinuses	Hardwood furniture manufacturers
**	Nasal sinuses	Leather workers

* Certain compounds or oxidation states only.
** Causative agent not known.

From R. Doll and R. Peto, 1981. *The causes of cancer.* Oxford: Oxford University Press,
p. 1238. Slightly amended and reproduced by permission from the Oxford University
Press.

and estimating for each type the possible contribution of occupation. Such an approach avoids the more unreliable procedure of trying to make a quantitative estimate of the hazards associated with broad groups of occupations without any reliable knowledge of the quantity of carcinogen to which employees are actually exposed. Through considering each cancer separately, Doll and Peto have estimated that 4% of all cancers are due to occupational factors. The calculation of this proportion is based principally on consideration of those cancers which can definitely result from occupational hazards. To this was added a token amount from cancers which possibly can be caused by occupational hazards (Doll & Peto, 1981, pp. 1242–1245).

Table 5.7 lists the types of cancer that definitely can be produced by occupational hazards and the proportion of deaths from each cause attributed to occupational factors for American males. The number of female cancer deaths attributed to occupation is less than one-seventh the number for males. By far the largest proportion of occupational cancer deaths is from lung cancer; 15% of all male lung cancers and 5% of all lung cancer in females. The most outstanding agent responsible for this is asbestos. It is estimated that asbestos may cause 5% of all present-day lung cancers and 1% or 2% of all cancer deaths. Occupational exposure to the combustion products of fossil fuels is also common (see Table 5.6). Although the relative risks from this exposure are seldom high, the number of workers exposed is considerable, such that another 5% of all male cases of lung cancer may be due to polycyclic hydrocarbons. Other recognized occupational causes of lung cancer have affected only small groups (Doll & Peto, 1981, pp. 1243–1244).

In the case of bladder cancer the proportion attributable to occupation can be estimated with more confidence than for other cancers, given the findings of prior research. Doll and Peto propose that 10% of cases of male bladder cancer and 5% in the case of females can be attributed to occupation. This would account for 831 of the bladder cancer deaths in the U.S. in 1978. Occupational leukemia deaths are probably responsible for 10% of male leukemia deaths and 5% in females. The proportions of the other cancers attributable to occupation have been based on interpretation of the literature and clinical impression, given the absence of firm evidence (Doll & Peto, 1981, pp. 1243–1244).

From this analysis asbestos and polycyclic hydrocarbons are by far the most important occupational causes of cancer. Asbestos is

TABLE 5.7: Types of cancer that definitely can be produced by occupational hazards and the proportion of deaths from these cancers ascribed to occupational hazards, U.S. males, 1978

Type of Cancer	Total no. of deaths, males	Proportion of deaths ascribed to occupational hazards, males	
		No. ascribed	% ascribed
Lung*+	71,006	10,651	15
Leukemia	8,683	868	10
Bladder	6,771	677	10
Prostate	21,674	217	1
Pleura, nasal sinuses, remaining respiratory sites	857	214	25
Skin other than melanoma	1,061	106	10
Mesentery & peritoneum**	652	98	15
Liver* & intrahepatic bile ducts	1,812	72	4
Larynx	2,909	58	2
Bone*	997	40	4
Other and unspecified cancers	15,445	1,045	7
Total	131,867		

* Includes many misdiagnosed secondary cancers from other sites.
** Also includes cancer of "unspecified digestive sites."
+ Assumed to include some miscertified cases of pleural mesothelioma.

From R. Doll and R. Peto, 1981. *The Causes of Cancer.* Oxford: Oxford University Press, p. 1244. Slightly amended and reproduced by permission from Oxford University Press.

also responsible for a specific form of pulmonary fibrosis which causes progressive disability and death. Despite these facts the epidemiology of asbestos-induced disease is only incompletely understood. In addition to the general methodological difficulties in assessing causation (see Chapter 4), diseases due to asbestos present their own special problems. Whereas exposure to asbestos in many early epidemiological studies was measured in terms of dust concentration, it is now recognized that the fiber concentration is the appropriate measure of dosage. This makes the interpretation of many studies difficult. Furthermore, the variable toxicity of different types of asbestos fiber, and the fact that industrial processes mix fibers, make the appropriate assessment of exposure even more complex. Both the carcinogenic and fibrosis-inducing effects of asbestos are enhanced by smoking (Hammond, Selikoff, & Seidman, 1979). In spite of these issues an acceptable degree of certitude can be given to a number of aspects of asbestosis-related diseases. In a review of studies in 22 working populations, all but one showed a dose-response relationship between asbestos exposure and lung cancer; the mortality ratios ranged from 0.77 to 7.6. This dose-response relationship is probably linear. With regard to asbestosis a dose-response relationship with exposure to asbestos is well established. Asbestos also causes mesothelioma and probably increases the incidence of laryngeal and gastrointestinal cancer (Shannon, 1982).

The epidemiological evidence concerning the role of occupational exposure to polycyclic aromatic hydrocarbons in causing lung cancer is only suggestive. Whereas increased risks have been observed in some occupational groups (Doll et al., 1972; Palmer & Scott, 1981), the risk for some groups in the same industry is small (Gibson, Martin, and Lockington, 1977). Uncertainty remains as to whether or not the observed increases in lung cancer are due to exposure to polycyclic aromatic hydrocarbons. However, it has been observed that products of combustion are associated with cancer ever since scrotal cancer was described in chimney sweeps over 200 years ago. The experimental carcinogenicity of certain pure polycyclic hydrocarbons is accepted without disagreement (Falk, Kotin & Mehler, 1964). Similarly, occupational skin cancers are closely related to contact with pitch and tar (Henry, 1947).

While occupation is a well-recognized cause of disease this usually applies to specific work populations which are small in size. In terms of mortality the contribution of occupation is small relative to life style. While its effect on morbidity is not well substantiated, this is possibly quite extensive.

Pollution

General environmental pollution results from both industrial and other sources, most of which are due to fuel combustion and industrial processes. The major pollutants include particulate matter, sulphur oxides, carbon monoxide, nitrogen dioxide, photochemical oxidants, and the hydrocarbons. The concentration of these substances in the environment is determined by the amount produced as well as by the rate of their removal by wind, rain, and currents. The resultant pollution may affect water, land, or air.

Water pollution can have a major effect on animal life, and in turn can affect humans, such as occurred in Japan when the industrial discharge of mercury into the sea was ingested by shellfish that were subsequently eaten. Bacterial contamination of water is a major health problem in those parts of the world without effective sewerage and water systems. Land pollution is often focal such as in the cases of industrial dumps and leaks from nuclear reactors. These forms of pollution can produce high exposures, but only to small groups, so their health effects on the community at large are thought to be small.

Air pollution, by contrast, usually involves a far wider exposure than either water or land pollution. The adverse effect of intense episodes of atmospheric pollution are well documented. In the London fog of December 1952, for example, there were 4,000 more deaths than usually occur at that time of the year. The deaths were mainly among infants and the elderly, and were due to the major respiratory diseases, coronary disease, and myocardial degeneration. The interpretation of such events is that the harmful effect of gross air pollution is to exacerbate existing disease and to hasten death among individuals with cardiac and respiratory disorders (McKeown & Lowe, 1966, pp. 156–157). The effects of low levels of air pollution are less well understood (Doll, 1978; Ferris, 1978).

Indirect evidence suggesting that long-term air pollution is harmful comes from rural–urban comparisons of mortality. Death rates from bronchitis, cancer of the lung, pneumonia, and respiratory tuberculosis increase with mounting population density. This ranges from the lowest level of mortality from these causes in rural areas, through towns, to the highest mortality in large urban conurbations (very large urban areas where one city runs into another without an intervening low density settlement) (McKeown & Lowe, 1966, pp. 51–52). The precise investigation of the health effects of low levels of air pollution faces a number of methodological difficulties relating to the identification of the active agent, measurement of the level of pollutant, interaction between pollutants, and controlling for confounding variables (Ferris, 1978).

In the case of sulphur oxides and particulates it is not justified to infer that the usual levels measured in the atmosphere have an effect on mortality. There is general consistency among a number of prospective studies concerning morbidity. Short-term effects of exposure to elevated levels of sulphur oxides and particulates include an increase in respiratory symptoms in patients with chronic bronchitis, reduced respiratory function ($FEV_{1.0}$), and an increase in frequency of asthma attacks (Ferris, 1978). The long-term effects of exposure include increased phlegm production (Fletcher et al., 1976, p. 272), increased respiratory disease, decreased respiratory function, and increased respiratory symptoms. Particulates are probably more important than the gaseous SO_2 in these associations (Ferris, 1978; Ferris et al., 1976).

Concern that air pollution may be responsible for cancer first arose when it was observed that urban rates of lung cancer were almost invariably greater than in rural areas. Many of the substances listed in Table 5.7 escape into the atmosphere. Those that escape in the greatest amounts are polycyclic hydrocarbons, arsenic, asbestos, and radioactive elements. These substances acting alone can only be responsible for a small number of cases. The mortality rate from lung cancer among nonsmokers is extremely low, irrespective of the area in which they live. Doll (1978) has estimated that in the absence of cigarette smoking the combined effect of all atmospheric carcinogens is not responsible for more than 5 cases of lung cancer per 100,000 persons per year in European populations. (The mortality rate from lung cancer for smokers of 1 to 9 cigarettes per day is 37:100,000.) Concerning the incidence of all cancer due to all forms of pollution, Doll and Peto (1981, p. 1251) have assigned the proportion of 2%, mainly because of the uncertain effect of combustion products of fossil fuels in urban air.

In summary, the documented impact of pollution on health is small with the effect on mortality being less than that on morbidity. However, the general inadequacy of the information on which this conclusion is based and the growing production of new chemical substances do not allow for complacency.

The Man-Made Environment

The third aspect of the environment to consider is that which human beings have specifically designed and constructed for themselves: walkways, rooms, houses, neighborhoods, cities, and planned living areas for work and recreation. Today the man-made environment is extremely complex. This is reflected in our limited understanding of how it affects our health. With respect to its influence on health, the designed environment has been studied at different levels, encompassing its esthetic qualities, the design of passageways, housing, the structure of neighborhoods, and comparison of the urban and rural environments.

The esthetic qualities of our surroundings, such as their beauty and naturalness, have been studied in terms of their effect on psychological well-being using quasi-experimental methods. In two trials, a positive association was found between the beauty of a room and the perception of energy and well-being. This effect was sustained over repeated exposures (Maslow & Mintz, 1956; Mintz, 1956). The emotional feelings invoked by scenes of natural landscape have been found to differ from those engendered by urban scenes (Ulrich, 1979). These laboratory studies and others (Griffin, Mauritzen, & Kasmar, 1969) demonstrate that perceptions and feelings can be affected by the esthetic nature of the environment.

The immediate physical environment also affects behavior. Design features such as room size and seating arrangements influence communication by affecting speed of reading, intensity of speaking, and social interaction (Griffin, Mauritzen, & Kasmar, 1969). Mobility and communication for the physically handicapped is particularly important to the quality of life. The architecture of ramps, doorways, corridors, open spaces, telephones, kitchens, and bathrooms, for example, all affect the ability of the disabled to perform specific functional activities. The relevance of any given aspect of architecture depends upon the type of physical handicap (Steinfeld et al, 1976).

In a review of housing and health, Cassell (1977) identifies that the literature is conflictual and that methodological limitations cloud the interpretation of many studies. There are, however, many direct effects of housing on health. These include lead poisoning due to peeling lead paint, accidents due to dilapidated structures, the physical effects of a lack of heating, and the infective illnesses associated with infestations and ineffective waste disposal (Last, 1980). In a classic study of apartment life and health, Fanning (1967) compared the health of women and children of similar social class in 398 apartments and 160 houses in a British air force base in Germany. Consultations to the general practitioner, referrals to specialists, the incidence of bronchitis, pneumonia, menstrual irregularities, and psychoneurotic disorders were all significantly higher among apartment dwellers. Only low back pain was more frequent in women in houses. While the frequency of illness differed, its severity was similar for the two groups. These differences varied with age, affecting mainly children under 10, women over 40 years of age, and those in their twenties. In a case-control study of nonfatal pedestrian accidents in Belfast, Backett and Johnston (1959) observed that children without a garden, yard, or playroom at home and those who did not play in protected areas were at an increased risk of a pedestrian accident. In much of the literature it is postulated that housing, and the man-made environment in general, exert their influence on health indirectly through promoting behavior which predisposes the individual to illness or accidents (Kasl, 1977).

Studies of neighborhood design and health also present inconsistent findings (Kasl, 1977). In one review concerning the elderly (Brody, 1977), a number of environmental factors were identified which probably influence well-being and physical function. Among these are proximity to friends and family, community resources, availability of appropriate transport, a physically safe environment, and spacial opportunities for socialization. In a prospective study in Baltimore (Wilner et al., 1962), the health effects of moving from a slum area to good housing were studied. Significant improvements occurred in physical health in the families who moved compared with those who remained in the slum, particularly in terms of the occurrence of accidents in individuals under 35 years of age.

The most extensively documented association of health and the man-made environment is the urban–rural distribution of injuries and causes of death. Although mortality from respiratory disease and lung cancer is higher in cities than the country (McKeown & Lowe, 1966, pp. 62–64), the design of cities probably has little to do directly with this. On the other hand, the lower death rates from road and work accidents in cities may be more closely related to structural differences between the two environments. While cities are safer in terms of the risk of accidental deaths, all nonwork injuries, particularly among the young, are more frequent in cities (Ford, 1976, pp. 55–63).

Although the literature on the health effects of the man-made environment is more limited than for any other broad category of risk factor some important conclusions can be made. The incidence of a number of illnesses, some attitudes, aspects of physical well-being, and the incidence and severity of accidents in given sectors of society all can be associated with the structure of the environment. These associations are not uniform throughout the community, but have a pattern of distribution in which a given health problem tends to occur in one age group in a particular environment. An obvious example is the exacerbation of physical immobility in the disabled when faced with inappropriate doorways and staircases. Other examples include the higher rate of psychoneurotic disorders in women over 40 years in apartments, and the high rate of nonwork-related accidents in young people in cities. Such evidence suggests that the effect of the physical environment is specific to identifiable at-risk groups.

A second point is the confounding influence of behavior. In at least two well-controlled studies it was observed that the use of community recreational facilities did not depend upon the availability of physical facilities. Among apartment dwellers and house dwellers with similar access to playgrounds, the apartment dwellers made less use of these facilities (Fanning, 1967). Children involved in pedestrian road accidents differed from control children in where they played despite comparable access to home and neighborhood recreational facilities (Backett & Johnston, 1959). On the basis of such findings it has been proposed that the man-made environment influences health through its effect on behavior (Kasl, 1977). This implies, therefore, that research should focus on behavior and specific health outcomes in particular at-risk groups and upon the man-made environment and its effect on behavior.

SUMMARY

The causes of disease have been described under the discrete headings of heredity, behavior, and environment. In contrast to diseases of previous centuries, the environment appears to be playing a small role relative to life style. While behavior is clearly the major determinant of modern diseases, heredity may be the major determinant of an individual's susceptibility to disease. Of all aspects of heredity and disease the role of genes in determining an individual's predisposition to chronic disease is the least understood.

In many aspects of lifestyle our knowledge is inadequate to provide a clear guide to developing healthy behavior. This is particularly the case with diet. In numerous instances people choose an "unhealthy" life style despite knowledge of its harmful effects. Beyond an understanding of the determinants of disease, it is necessary to understand how to change behavior in order to benefit from new knowledge. Concerning lifestyle in particular, it is not as though the changes required are discrete activities; rather, multiple facets of everyday life need to be modified. It has become necessary, therefore, to understand the interaction of the many aspects of modern behavior in determining the major chronic diseases such as heart disease and cancer. This is the focus of the next chapter.

Chapter **6**

Risks III: Selected Diseases and Their Causes

With disorders such as those caused by a single gene, a chromosomal aberration, or an infection, the relationship between the causative factor and the disease is readily identifiable and is highly specific. These diseases can be attributed to a single cause. The etiology of the majority of chronic diseases is quite different. Cancer and heart disease, for example, result from multiple factors, each of which usually has a relatively weak relationship with the disease. In the case of smoking and lung cancer, a causative relationship which is particularly well documented, the majority of smokers do not die of lung cancer. A new and distinctive approach needs to be taken in order to understand the cause of chronic disease. The purpose of this chapter is to summarize the evidence concerning the etiology of the two major chronic diseases, cancer and heart disease, and to define the relative importance of their various risk factors.

CANCER

The understanding of the causes of cancer has come from both epidemiological and laboratory research. The biological mechanisms whereby a normal cell develops into a cancer cell is a vital component of our knowledge. This information defines the stages in the process that follow exposure to the cause of cancer and which precede its clinical manifestation. This is the contribution of biological or mechanistic research. Throughout life human beings are exposed to a plethora of external factors, some of which are harmful. Epidemiological research endeavors to identify the factors that either cause cancer or protect against it. With these two dimensions in mind the development of cancer can be thought of as having both an environmental history, during which a person is exposed to cancer producing agents, and a biological history, involving the growth and development of the malignancy. The nature of the biological and epidemiological evidence, on which current knowledge is based, will be discussed before considering each of the major causes of cancer.

Evidence Concerning the Cause of Cancer

Biological Evidence

A cancer develops from a single cell. This occurs when a cell is no longer subject to the normal biological controls that are responsible for maintaining the equilibrium in the body's population of 10 million cells. Cells are dividing throughout life to replace those that are lost or destroyed. However, organs differ in terms of their frequency of normal cell divisions and this relates to the occurrence of cancer. Cells in gut, skin, and bone marrow multiply continuously throughout life and are the sites of many common cancers. In the liver, thyroid, and other glands, cells seldom multiply in adult life, although they can if needed to do so and they can become cancerous. Nerve cells, on the other hand, do not multiply in mature tissue, and cancers of nerve cells are found only in infants (Cairns, 1978, pp. 16–17).

The growth of a cancer starts with an abnormality in a single cell, and the essential property of the cancer cell is that it creates an expanding population of cells like itself. In this sense cancer is a form of hereditary disease. The process of inheritance or lineage is therefore fundamental to understanding the difference between a normal collection of apparently similar cells, such as those in one lobe of the liver, and a cancer. An organ such as the liver does not arise from a single cell, but is a mosaic made up of descendents from several different families of cells that originate early in embryonic development, when the embryo consists of no more than 20 cells (Cairns, 1978, pp. 17–20).

Normal cells are programmed to follow a set pattern of behavior. For example, the epidermal cells of skin are usually 5 to 10 cells thick. The round cells in the basal layer divide to produce new cells which are programmed to differentiate into flat squamous cells and then fuse and die to form keratin flakes. The only cells to divide are the basal cells; these cells grow out to the surface and respect the boundary set by the basement membrane. When a carcinoma develops, the basal cells fail to differentiate, and they die as normal epidermal cells do. They no longer respect their territorial boundary, but grow through the basement membrane, invading the underlying dermis (Cairns, 1978, pp. 24–27). In order to understand this change in cell behavior, it is necessary to understand something of the chemical basis of heredity.

The behavior and structure of a cell are determined by the proteins produced by the cell. The characteristics of these proteins are defined by their amino acid sequence. It is the primary function of the deoxyribonucleic acid (DNA) in the cell nucleus to dictate this amino acid sequence. The instructions for this are contained in the genetic code of the DNA as defined by the sequences of its own building bricks or nucleotide bases, of which there are only four types. DNA consists of a pair of unbranching chains of bases (adenine, thymine, guanine, and cytosine), coupled together with adenine always opposite thymine, and guanine opposite cytosine. When the cell divides, the DNA is replicated and its sequence of bases is faithfully copied and handed to the next generation. Likewise, any change in the sequence of bases, a mutation, is inherited from one generation to the next (Cairns, 1978, pp. 70–78).

Many agents interact with DNA to cause mutations. Radiation can damage DNA, and chemical agents have a wide range of effects, such as removing side groups from bases, adding new chemical groups, and even linking themselves onto DNA (e.g., the polycyclic hydrocarbon benzpyrene becomes linked to guanine). When germ cells in the testis or ovary are affected, the level of deleterious mutations in the offspring is raised. Birth defects can occur when developmental errors result from mutations in somatic cells of the fetus, and it is thought that when mutations affect somatic cells in adult life they can cause cancer (Cairns, 1978, p. 85). So many known carcinogens have proved also to be powerful mutagens that it seems almost certain that most forms of cancer are due at least in part to changes in DNA. However, very little is known of the functions of genes which need to be mutated in order to develop cancer. Despite our lack of knowledge, the study of carcinogens has added to our understanding of the role of mutation in the development of cancer (Cairns, 1978, p. 90).

Agents which induce neoplastic changes include physical, chemical, and biologic agents. Radiation is the principal physical carcinogen. Biologic agents include viruses and parasites. Originally it was thought that the metabolism of chemical carcinogens destroyed their potency; it is now recognized that metabolism is a critical factor in their effectiveness. A large number of chemical carcinogens are initially inactive, from which state they are metabolized in the host to an active ultimate form. It is thought that the critical site of action of the ultimate forms of chemical carcinogens is DNA (Pitot, 1979).

A prominent feature of carcinogenesis is the long lapse in time between the initial exposure to a carcinogen and the appearance of cancer. For example, lung cancer rates do not start to rise until approximately 20 years following onset of smoking. Knowing why this long delay occurs is fundamental to understanding why a cell turns malignant. In some instances the process of carcinogenesis can be separated into two stages—initiation and promotion. Initiation probably involves mutation due to a carcinogen binding to DNA. Promotion is less well understood but all recognized promoters have in common the one feature of provoking increased cell multiplication. Experimentally, a cancer results only when the application of the promoter follows the initiator. The reverse order of application does not result in cancer (Cairns, 1978, pp. 90–94). The idea that there are separate steps driven by separate factors has important implications for prevention. If an intermediate step can be identified it might be possible to interrupt the process and prevent the ultimate development of cancer. For example, in the case of carcinoma of the cervix, the diagnosable abnormalities of dysplasia and carcinoma in situ look very much like the successive stages in a sequence lasting decades, which are sometimes followed by a fully invasive cancer (Barron & Richart, 1970; Cairns, 1978, pp. 147, 149). On the basis of the prevalence of initiating agents in our environment in the form of air pollution, diet, drugs, and radiation, among others, it is quite likely that initiation of neoplastic cells is a frequent event, and it may be that the critical step in the development of cancer is that of promotion (Pitot, 1979).

As a final point concerning biological evidence it is relevant to consider the variability in the characteristics of cancers. Epithelial tissues (e.g., skin, respiratory tract, gut, the lining of breast, pancreas, and thyroid) are responsible for more than 90% of all human cancers. Less than 10% arise from supporting tissues and circulating cells. In all, more than 200 distinct varieties of cancer have been recognized; however, nearly half of all deaths are due to cancers of the lung, bowel, and breast (Cairns, 1978, pp. 20–22). Cancers of different origin behave differently. Basal cell carcinoma does not metastasize, whereas cancer of the neighboring melanocyte metastasizes rapidly. Metastatic cells from different origins tend to establish secondary cancers in different organs; for example, lung cancer metastasizes to the brain while cancer of the breast and prostate metastasize to bone. There is also considerable variation in cancers originating from the same type of organ. In the case of breast cancer, the tumor may arise in epithelium, stroma, duct tissue, or alveolar tissue or it may be quite undifferentiated so its exact origin is unidentifiable (Cairns, 1978, pp. 120–128).

The biology of cancer has contributed considerably to understanding the cause of cancer as well as the potential of prevention. Cancer appears to result from environmental exposure to a wide variety of agents which interfere with the molecular control of cell function. This occurs in a stepwise fashion over a prolonged period of time. The diversity in the types and characteristics of cancer corresponds with the variety in the structure and function of the cells in which cancer occurs. Cancer is not a simple phenomenon, but represents a broad category of diseases containing many different types of malignancy, each of which has its own particular characteristics. This variation between cancers, which is so apparent in the biology of neoplasia, has played an important part in facilitating the investigation of the epidemiology of cancer.

Epidemiological Evidence

The major contribution of epidemiology to the understanding of cancer has been through the identification of environmental factors associated with cancer and by describing groups of individuals at increased risk of malignancy. The evidence that has contributed to these findings has come mainly from observations of four types: observations of differences in incidence between communities and groups, changes in incidence on migration and over time, and identification of many specific causes and preventive factors.

The comparison of groups is the basis of the epidemiologic method. Evidence that cancer is due to avoidable environmental factors has accumulated over the last half-century from observations of differences in cancer rates between a variety of communities. International comparisons of specific cancers show dramatic differences in incidence (total cancer rates vary a lot less). Doll and Peto (1981, pp. 1198–1200) have reported on an international comparison of 19 common types of cancer which are both reliably recorded and are common enough somewhere to affect at least 1% of men or women. In all of these cancers the variation in incidence was considerable, in all instances differing at least six-fold and sometimes more than 100-fold. These included cancers in the major sites of the gastrointestinal, respiratory, and repro-ductive systems as well as cancer of the skin, bladder, liver, pancreas, and breast. Cancer of the lung was 35 times greater in England than Nigeria, colon cancer 10 times greater in Mozambique than England, and skin cancer more than 200 times greater in Queensland than Bombay. Evidence has also come from differences in cancer rates between religious groups such as Seventh-day Adventists and the general population (Phillips, 1975), and differences between educational groups (Lilienfeld, Levin, & Kessler, 1972, pp. 215–232).

A second category of epidemiological evidence comes from studies of the change in cancer incidence with migration. Studies of cancer among Japanese living in Japan, Hawaii, and California show large differences in cancer rates. Among Japanese in Japan stomach cancer is far higher, and colon, breast, and prostate cancer are considerably lower, than among Japanese immigrants in the United States (Buell & Dunn, 1965; Doll & Peto, 1981, p. 1201). Other examples include lower rates of liver cancer among black Americans than occur in Nigeria, the fall in oral cancer among Indians who migrated to Fiji and South Africa, and the high rates of skin cancer acquired by British immigrants to Fiji (Doll & Peto, 1981, pp. 1200–1201). These observations strengthen the case in favor of cancer being environmentally determined, and detract considerably from any suggestion that the international differences in cancer are genetically based on racial characteristics.

Changes in the rates of particular cancers over time within a population of which the genetic pool is reasonably constant are conclusive evidence that external factors are responsible. Observations of such secular changes in cancer are subject to biases due to changing diagnostic methods and criteria, recording stand-ards, and generally improved medical knowledge. After taking into account the effect of such measurement errors there are a number of changes in cancer rates which clearly have resulted from altered environmental factors. These include the increase in esophageal cancer in the black population of South Africa, the continuing increase in lung cancer throughout most of the world, the increase in pleural mesothelioma in males in industrialized countries, and the decrease in cancer of the tongue in Britain and in cancer of the cervix and stomach throughout Western Europe and North America (Cairns, 1978, pp. 42–46; Doll & Peto, 1981, pp. 1201–1202).

The most direct evidence of avoidable environmental factors causing cancer is experimental evidence. As scientific experiments of suspected carcinogens are restricted to animals the most direct evidence comes mainly from occupational exposures and cohort studies of cancer rates following the removal of a suspected carcinogen. This category of epidemiological evidence has been discussed in detail in Chapter 5.

Although the combination of biological and epidemiological evidence has disclosed a great deal about the cause of cancer, there remains much to be learned. We are all well aware of the number of deaths due to cancer. Out of the many components of the environment a number of carcinogens have been identified accurately. The relationship between these two sets of information is imprecisely understood. In order to set priorities it is necessary to know the proportion of cancers for which each cause is responsible. Not enough is known to allow a direct quantitative estimate of the cancer risk attributable to each known carcinogen. Where adequate data are available, Doll and Peto (and others before them) have made quantitative estimates and otherwise "have made estimates on the basis of extrapolations of uncertain reliability, clinical impressions and contemporary hypotheses" (Doll & Peto, 1981, p. 1220). Their work is the basis for the following description of the causes of cancer.

Avoidable Causes of Cancer

On the basis of the evidence in this and the previous chapter, cancer is determined principally by environmental factors. These factors are largely under our control. For this reason, and because the prime interest in studying cancer is to avoid its occurrence, this section is limited to the avoidable causes of cancer. In considering each cause Doll and Peto's estimate is given of the proportion of all cancer attributable to the given cause.

Tobacco

No other single factor is responsible for more cancer than tobacco. The major impact on cancer of reduction in smoking or in using tobacco in a less harmful way would be upon the incidence of lung cancer. By late middle age lung cancer among regular smokers is more than 10 times greater than among lifelong nonsmokers. There would be benefit also in the rates of cancer of the mouth, pharynx, larynx, esophagus, bladder, and probably pancreas and possibly kidney (Doll & Peto, 1981, pp. 1220-1221). The evidence that cigarette smoking is a direct cause of cancer comes from many epidemiological sources as well as animal experiments (Department of Health, Education and Welfare, 1979). Selected studies are reviewed in Chapter 5.

The proportion of all cancer in the United States attributable to smoking has been calculated by estimating separately the number of deaths from each type of cancer caused by smoking. The chief sources of data used were: (1) male and female age-specific death rates from each cancer among Americans in 1978; (2) the corresponding death rates from a control group of half a million Americans who said they never smoked regularly and who were followed prospectively between 1959 and 1972 (Garfinkel, 1980); and (3) some approximate information about national smoking habits. In this way Doll and Peto (1981, pp. 1221–1224) estimated that in 1978, 30% of all cancer deaths were due to smoking, and by the mid-1980s this proportion probably will have increased to at least 33%.

Diet

Diet is probably no less important than smoking as a cause of cancer; however, the evidence is mainly indirect. For the purposes of this section diet refers only to those items that occur in natural food or are produced during the natural processes of storage, cooking, or digestion. Even with this restricted definition, the variety in the composition and use of food makes this subject complex and difficult to investigate.

Five possible ways in which diet may induce cancer will be considered. The first is overnutrition. Marked reductions in the incidence of naturally occurring tumors have resulted from dietary restriction in animal experiments (Jose, 1979). Humans who are overweight are also at increased risk of some cancers. The one most definitely related to overnutrition is carcinoma of the endometrium, for which the mortality ratio in the most obese increases to 5.4 (Lew & Garfinkel, 1979). Because this disease can be produced by excess exposure to estrogen, the occurrence in the obese has been explained by the fact that adrenal hormones in adipose tissue are the only natural source of estrogens postmenopausally (Armstrong, 1977). Important associations between overnutrition and cancer have also been observed with cancer of the gall bladder in females and with cancer of the cervix (Lew & Garfinkel, 1979). Colorectal cancer and breast cancer are generally associated with a high standard of living in adult life and have been suspected to be due to diets high in fat and meat (in the case of colorectal cancer). Overnutrition and breast cancer can be linked in an additional way. A high standard of nutrition in childhood advances the age of menarche, and early menarche is associated with an increase in the risk of breast cancer (Doll & Peto, 1981, 1233–1235).

A second mechanism is by ingestion of powerful, direct-acting carcinogens or their precursors. Carcinogens may exist in natural foodstuffs, such as in bracken fern, which is associated with a three fold increase in risk of carcinoma of the esophagus among Japanese who eat it compared with those who do not (Hirayama, 1979). Carcinogens can be produced during cooking. Benzo[a]pyrene and other polycyclic hydrocarbons can be produced by pyrolysis when meat or fish are broiled or smoked or when any food is fried in fat that is used repeatedly. Recently it has been recognized that during storage, microorganisms can produce carcinogens. It is now thought that aflatoxins, produced by a fungus which contaminates peanuts and other carbohydrate foods in hot and humid climates, are a major factor in liver cancer in some tropical countries (Doll & Peto, 1981, pp. 1227–1228).

Carcinogens such as nitroso compounds can be produced in the gut and urinary bladder, providing the appropriate substrate and conditions exist. Nitrosable compounds occur naturally in many foods, particularly fish and meat. Their formation requires a mildly acid medium or bacterial assistance and is assisted by formaldehyde or thiocyanate ions (possibly from tobacco smoke). This process is inhibited by antioxidants such as vitamin C. There are therefore many ways in which carcinogenic nitroso compounds might be formed and many factors that may affect their production. It is not known whether the amounts produced correlate with the incidence of particular types of cancer (Doll & Peto, 1981, pp. 1228–1229).

A fourth way in which diet may influence the occurrence of cancer is by its effect on transportation, activation, or deactivation of carcinogens. For example, if some component of dietary fiber reduces the incidence of colorectal cancer, several mechanisms for this can be proposed. This may occur as a result of the decreased time stools remain in the bowel, or because of the reduced concentration of carcinogens in the stool. Alternatively, the concentration or nature of bacteria in the bowel may be changed, some of which may produce or destroy carcinogenic metabolites. Many carcinogens require chemical activation by oxidation, peroxidation, or by the generation of short-lived intermediates before they become carcinogenic. The dangers of some of these carcinogens could potentially be reduced if the appropriate parts of the body were permeated with substances which interfere with the chemical activation of carcinogens. β-carotene, found in carrots and some other vegetables, is one such substance. From a number of studies there is indication of some protective effect of β-carotene in the diet and blood (Peto et al., 1981).

Finally, diet may influence cancer rates by affecting the promotion of cells in which a carcinogenic change has already been initiated. Vitamin A in experimental animals can reduce the probability that affected cells advance to tumor cells; and in human studies circulating vitamin A appears to protect against cancer (Doll & Peto, 1981, pp. 1232–1233; Kark et al., 1981; Wald et al., 1980).

From these five mechanisms the complexity of the relationship of diet and cancer is readily apparent. Many mechanisms have not been mentioned. Although it may not be possible to prevent exposure to dietary carcinogens, it may be feasible to employ dietary factors in an indirect fashion. Particularly, it may be possible to prescribe protective dietary strategies which inhibit tumor development despite exposure to carcinogens. Doll and Peto (1981, p. 1235) have estimated that 35% of all cancers may be avoidable through dietary means although they make no claim as to the reliability of this figure. The proportion of specific cancers which they consider could possibly be reduced through changes to diet are stomach and bowel, 90%; endometrium, gall bladder, pancreas, and breast, 50%; lung, larynx, bladder, cervix, mouth, pharynx, and esophagus, 20%; and other types of cancer, 10%. Based on these estimates, diet and smoking combined cause 65% of cancers. Compared with this the individual contribution of each of the remaining causes, of which there are many, is only small.

Alcohol

Alcohol alone probably plays little part in causing cancer. Its effect is probably to facilitate contact between extrinsic carcinogens and the stem cells lining the larynx and the upper digestive tract. The estimated 3% of cancers attributed to alcohol, described in Chapter

5, is based on the combined effect of interaction of alcohol and smoking. Most of these cancers could be avoided by the absence of smoking even with continued alcohol consumption. This proportion has not been counted in the cancers attributed to smoking (Doll & Peto, 1981, pp. 1224–1225).

Food Additives

While food additives are a potential source of carcinogens, probably less than 1% of cancers can be attributed to them. In the case of saccharin, animal experiments indicate it is a weak carcinogen but epidemiological studies show no association with cancer. On the other hand, nitrites used to preserve meats are additives that would need to be held responsible for some cases of cancer if the formation of nitrosamines and nitrosamides proves to be important in producing intestinal cancer (Doll & Peto, 1981, pp. 1235–1237).

Reproductive and Sexual Behavior

The role of reproductive behavior in causing cancer has been described previously in Chapter 5. It is estimated that 7% of cancers, principally cancers of the breast, ovary, endometrium, and cervix, could be avoided through modification of reproductive behavior (Doll & Peto, 1981, pp. 1237–1238).

Occupation

Likewise, occupation has been considered in detail already. Doll and Peto (1981, pp. 1238–1245) estimate that 4% of avoidable cancer is due to occupation.

Pollution

In the case of the effects of pollution, described in Chapter 5, a token figure of 2% has been assigned to the proportion of cancers due to avoidable sources of pollution. This percentage is based principally on the estimated effect of the combustion products of fossil fuels in urban air (Doll & Peto, 1981, pp. 1245–1251).

Industrial Products

Industrial products such as paints, plastics, dyes, polishes, solvents, detergents, cosmetics, and fabrics are too numerous to list. There is inadequate laboratory and human evidence to know if some of these products are harmful or truly harmless. Current trends in cancer incidence do not indicate that the huge increase in synthetic chemicals since World War II has had harmful effects. Despite this, caution in interpretation is warranted. If a cancer epidemic due to industrial products was to occur this would not appear until at least 20 years following initial exposure. The rapid growth in synthetic chemicals dates mainly from the late 1950s so that a resultant rise in cancer would not yet be apparent (Davis & Magee, 1979). Based on current cancer rates less than 1% of cancers have been estimated as resulting from industrial products (Doll & Peto, 1981, p. 1251).

Medicines and Medical Procedures

Of the known carcinogens many have been used in medical practice. These include cyclophosphamide, melphalan, arsenic, busulfan, chlornaphazine, immunosuppressive drugs, ionizing radiations, estrogens, phenacetin, polycyclic hydrocarbons, oxymetholone, steroid contraceptives, and ultraviolet light. Some of these treatments have limited use or are prescribed for patients with a reduced life expectancy, so their net effect on cancer incidence is small. Others, however, such as ionizing radiations, estrogens, and steroid contraceptives, are used very widely. It is estimated that approximately one half of 1% of cancers are attributable to the medical use of ionizing radiation. Estrogens probably contribute to both endometrial and breast cancer. In the case of oral contraceptives it is thought that the number of cancers caused is very small. In sum, therefore, the proportion of cancers due to medical practice has been estimated at 1%, one half of which is due to ionizing radiations (Doll & Peto, 1981, pp. 1252-1253).

Geophysical Factors

In contrast to most other causes of cancer, the number of cancer deaths attributable to naturally occurring ionizing irradiation and ultraviolet light is quite reliably known. About 3% of cancer deaths are due to geophysical factors. Only a proportion of this is avoidable, so that no more than 2% of cancer deaths are due to geophysical factors and are avoidable (Doll & Peto, 1981, pp. 1253-1254).

Infection

While it is well established that cancer is not an infectious disease, viruses, bacteria, and parasites do contribute to the occurrence of cancer. Viruses interfere with cellular DNA and can contribute directly to the biological process of carcinogenesis. Bacteria and parasites can influence neoplasia in other ways, including the production and destruction of carcinogens and by facilitating the chemical conversion of substances to carcinogens. It is estimated that about 10% of cancers are attributable to infection, 5% from viruses and 5% from other infections. The contribution of infection may be much higher if infection leads to cancer in a number of indirect ways (Doll & Peto, 1981, pp. 1254–1255).

Discussion

The cause of cancer is a complex subject out of which no clear strategy for prevention has yet been defined. At the molecular level, the initiation of carcinogenesis appears to be a common event which can result from many factors—physical, chemical, and biological. The more important step in neoplasia development may be promotion, which starts a cell's malignant proliferation. In addition to carcinogenic factors in the environment there are factors which protect against malignancy. Of the causes of cancer, tobacco is the most important and the best understood in terms of its malignant effects. Diet, on the other hand, is probably of comparable importance, but the data on its epidemiological impact are much less reliable. In terms of factors which protect against cancer, these are not well understood, although β-carotene, vitamin A, and pentose fiber all exert some protection directly or indirectly. It is possible that an important contribution to the future prevention of cancer will come from the prescription of protective measures, whereas proscription of harmful factors or activities could prove unpopular and ineffective.

ISCHEMIC HEART DISEASE

Ischemic heart disease, like cancer, has a multifactorial etiology. Its epidemic rise in this century and the recent decline in heart disease deaths confirm the role of the environment in its causation. The focus of this section is principally, but not exclusively, on environmental risk factors. Similar to cancer, the best predictor of heart disease is age. There is also a large sex difference. In the case of heredity the relationship is quite unclear (Blackburn & Gillum, 1980). The hypothesis that susceptibility to arteriosclerosis in humans is genetically determined remains conjectural and a subject for further research. Animal experiments have provided supportive evidence for this hypothesis (Goldstein, Kita & Brown, 1983). A family history of heart disease can be partly explained in a proportion of cases by a familial lifestyle (American Heart Association, 1980), but the role of genes in these cases remains undefined. An occasional case of ischemic heart disease has an hereditary basis, but familial hyperlipoproteinemia is rare and accounts for a very small proportion of hyperlipidemia (Glueck, Mattson, & Bierman, 1978). In addition to the association with constitutional factors, such as age and sex, there is an important relationship between heart disease and some other diseases. The first part of this section deals with these diseases as well as the major modifiable risk factors. This is followed by consideration of the biological mechanisms that help explain how certain risk factors influence the pathogenesis of ischemic heart disease.

Risk Factors

Hypertension

The relationship of elevated blood pressure and coronary heart disease is well established and has been demonstrated repeatedly (Keys, 1980, pp. 103–120; Pooling Project Research Group, 1978; Stamler, 1979). In the Seven Countries Study (Keys, 1980, pp. 103–120, 321–323), the two characteristics that were most significant in predicting the onset of coronary heart disease were age and resting blood pressure. In the Finnish data of the study a systolic blood pressure of 150 mmHg in a 50-year-old man was associated with an 18% greater incidence of myocardial infarction or coronary death than a pressure of 140 mmHg at the same age. The importance of systolic blood pressure was no less than diastolic blood pressure. Median systolic blood pressure explained 47% of the variance in death rates from coronary heart disease, and diastolic pressure explained 42%.

Diabetes Mellitus and Hyperglycemia

Diabetics have an increased incidence of coronary heart disease that is independent of the control of hyperglycemia (Stamler et al., 1979). The risk for male diabetics is twice that for nondiabetics, and for females it is increased three times. The net effect of this is that the sex ratio in the incidence of coronary heart disease is not apparent in diabetics (Dawber, 1980, pp. 190–201). While the relationship between diabetes, arteriosclerosis, and coronary heart disease is well established, this association is poorly understood.

Smoking

The risk of coronary heart disease among smokers has been described in detail previously (Chapter 5). In the U.S. Veterans Study (Rogot & Murray, 1980) the mortality ratio for coronary disease among smokers was only 1.58, compared with 11.28 for lung cancer. Despite this, more than 50% of excess deaths due to smoking were coronary deaths because of the high prevalence of ischemic heart disease. Although it is well accepted that smoking is an important risk factor for coronary disease, this has not been observed in all studies. In the Seven Countries Study (Keys, 1980, pp. 325–327), for example, "coronary death rate or the coronary incidence rates of the cohorts could not be shown to be related to any measure of the smoking habits of the cohorts" (p. 325). Failure to find this association probably relates to a lack of comparability of the cohorts on other attributes related to coronary artery disease. The weight of evidence indicates that smoking is an important risk factor and that the risk of death from coronary disease increases with the number of cigarettes smoked (Doll & Peto, 1976; Pooling Project Research Group, 1978; Rogot & Murray, 1980).

Diet

Evidence of the diet–atherosclerosis relationship is extensive and complex, and includes notable inconsistencies (McGill, McMahon, & Wene, 1981). Nevertheless, our "rich" diet has been designated as "a *primary, essential and necessary cause* of the current epidemic of premature atherosclerotic disease raging in the Western industrialized countries. Cigarette smoking and hypertension are important secondary or complementary causes" (Stamler, 1978, p. 11). The data on which this statement is based came from a number of sources.

Animal experiments in nonhuman primates have shown that a sustained diet high in fat and cholesterol produces hypercholesterolemia, extensive atherosclerosis, and fatal myocardial infarction (Armstrong & Warner, 1971; Stamler, 1979). When this typical diet is replaced by one low in all fats, or low in saturated fat and cholesterol but containing unsaturated vegetable oils, the atherosclerotic lesions regress (Armstrong, 1976; Wissler, 1978). The addition of cholesterol to the diet of primates not only elevates serum cholesterol but also changes the distribution of cholesterol within the lipoprotein fraction. The rise is mainly in cholesterol carried by low-density lipoprotein (LDL), so that the ratio of LDL to high-density lipoprotein (HDL) increases (Mahley et al., 1978; Stamler, 1979).

Human postmortem studies have found the same relationship between diet and occlusive vascular disease. In the International Atherosclerosis Project (IAP) (McGill, 1968) the degree of atherosclerosis in over 31,000 persons who died in 15 cities throughout the world was analyzed in terms of diet and other variables. A strong correlation was found between the percentages of calories from total dietary fat and the occurrence of severe aortic and coronary atherosclerosis (McGill, 1968; Stamler, 1978).

In the Seven Countries Study (Keys, 1980, pp. 248–262, 333–335) over 12,000 men in Finland, Greece, Italy, Japan, The Netherlands, the United States, and Yugoslavia were studied prospectively. The relationship between diet and both the 10-year incidence and death rates from coronary heart disease were analyzed. Total dietary fat had a correlation of 0.39 with incidence and 0.50 with deaths from ischemic heart disease. Dietary saturated fat calories correlated highly with both incidence ($r=0.73$) and coronary deaths ($r=0.84$).

These findings are further supported by a number of migration studies in which increases in dietary fat on migration (and other lifestyle changes) are associated with coronary disease. It has also been shown through the systematic study of dietary trends and coronary disease mortality in different countries that an increase in heart disease deaths is occurring in countries where dietary fat and calories are increasing; this contrasts with the decline in coronary deaths in the United States, which is associated with a decline in the same risk factors (Stamler, 1978).

The deleterious effect of a fatty and "rich" diet on coronary heart disease seems indisputable on the basis of such studies as those above. However, in a number of well conducted epidemiological studies on culturally homogeneous groups only low-order or no correlations between diet and serum cholesterol and diet and heart disease have been found (Frank, Berenson, & Webber, 1978; Gleuck & Conner, 1978; Gordon, 1970; Nichols et al., 1976). These results are the basis for a divergence of opinion on the diet–heart relationship (Gleuck, Mattson, & Bierman, 1978; Mann, 1977). In these studies the unit of measurement is the individual and not a group (as in the international studies), and this is thought to be a major factor underlying their failure to identify a strong diet–cholesterol–heart disease association (Keys, 1980, p. 335; McGill, McMahon, & Wene, 1981). Various explanations for these different findings have been proposed, one of which is that intraindividual variation in diet is as great as variation between individuals. Despite the existence of these paradoxical findings the weight of evidence more probably favors diet being a major coronary heart disease risk factor.

In spite of the importance of diet in heart disease, difficulty in making an accurate clinical assessment of diet reduces its usefulness as an index of individual risk. Added to this is the wide variation in risk among individuals with a similar diet. For these reasons an easily measured biological variable such as serum cholesterol is of particular utility in clinical practice.

Serum Cholesterol

Serum cholesterol is the best single indicator of coronary heart disease risk (Stamler, 1981). It has been found consistently to relate to atherosclerosis and the incidence of ischemic heart disease (Gordon et al., 1974; Keys, 1980; McGill, 1968; Pooling Project Research Group, 1978). The relative risk of a major coronary event in the Pooling Project (1978) was two and one-half times as high for men with a serum cholesterol of 250–299 mg% compared with those with a level below 175 mg%. The relationship is apparently continuous without evidence of a critical level; however, above 240 mg% the risk of heart disease is approximately twice that for individuals with a serum cholesterol below this level. An inverse relationship has been found between HDL cholesterol and coronary heart disease (Gordon et al., 1977).

Both the incidence of coronary heart disease and mean levels and distributions of total serum cholesterol vary widely between populations (Keys, 1980, pp. 85–95, 121–135), while at birth in all countries the total serum cholesterol means and distributions are similar (Wynder et al., 1979). Among migrant populations, the mean and distribution of serum cholesterol approach the levels of the adopted country whether higher or lower than the country of origin (Marmot et al., 1975).

Other Factors

A number of other factors have also been considered cardiovascular risk factors. Physical exercise is one such variable that protects against a coronary event (see Chapter 5). Similarly, the increased risk of venous and arterial thrombotic episodes, including coronary occlusion, due to oral contraceptives is well established (Royal College of General Practitioners, 1977). Obesity, on the other hand, has been a suspected predisposing factor but with the exception of extreme obesity it has been shown that obesity is not an important risk factor for heart disease (Keys, 1980; pp. 166–195, 327–329).

Multiple Risk Factors

From among the multiple factors associated with coronary heart disease it has been found that hypertension, smoking, and serum cholesterol are the three most important and accurately measurable variables. No single causative agent has been identified. The effect of any one of these three major risk factors is to at least double the likelihood of a coronary event within the ensuing decade. When two or all of these factors are present together the risk is 4 or 5 times that of individuals in whom these factors are absent (Stamler, 1981). Even when all the major risk factors are present this provides only an incomplete estimate of the coronary disease burden of the population (Jenkins, 1976a). It is important to look beyond the above variables to find additional causes to heart disease.

Psychosocial Factors

It is possible that psychosocial factors play a part in the development of coronary heart disease and account for a proportion of the disease which cannot be fully explained by other risk factors. Many psychosocial variables have been studied in relation to heart disease, including socioeconomic status, education, marital status, religion, social mobility, anxiety, life problems, stress, coronary-prone behavior pattern, and acculturation (Jenkins, 1976a, 1976b). The results of this research are conflicting, and no definite relationships have been established with the probable exceptions of personality type and acculturation.

Coronary-prone behavior pattern or type A behavior has been studied extensively. This is characterized by intense striving, competitiveness, impatience, time urgency, abruptness, overcommitment to vocation, and excessive drive and hostility. In a review of 24 studies between 1970 and 1975, only one did not find an association between at least some of these behaviors and the occurrence of coronary disease (Jenkins, 1976b). In the Western Collaborative Group Study (Rosenman et al., 1975), over 8.5 years of follow-up, men with the coronary-prone behavior pattern had 1.7 to 4.5 times the rate of new coronary disease as men judged to have the opposite type of personality. The relative risk was higher for younger men. A historical prospective analysis of thousands of male and female Kaiser Permanente subscribers (Friedman et al., 1974) was the one study which did not show an association between type A behavior and coronary heart disease.

In the Ni-Hon-San study (Marmot & Syme, 1976) the effect of acculturation on coronary disease was investigated. Of the 3,809 Japanese-Americans in California who were studied, those most acculturated to Western culture had a 3- to 5-fold excess of coronary heart disease over Japanese-Americans who adhered to traditional Japanese customs. The importance of this study is that it establishes that some sociocultural factor(s) affect the occurrence of coronary disease. The protective effect may relate to the strong group cohesion and social stability that characterizes traditional Japanese society and that is lacking in the life style of coronary-prone behavior. This interpretation is consistent with the relationship between social networks and mortality found in the Alameda County Study (Berkman & Syme, 1979).

Discussion

Investigation of the etiology of coronary heart disease has presented repeated frustrations to the epidemiologist due to the significant yet small contributions to the disease made by multiple factors. No one factor is clearly the principal cause, although important associations have been found with hypertension, smoking, diet, serum cholesterol, diabetes, exercise, oral contraceptives, and some psychosocial factors. It is possible that from among this list of risk factors one such as diet will ultimately be shown to be the major cause of heart disease. At present, the identification of the precise role of diet is hampered by methodological difficulties such as imprecision in the measurement of an individual's diet and the large variability in dietary behavior. Epidemiological research has contributed much to understanding the relationship between life style and heart disease, and there have also been important advances made in elucidating the biological changes which occur in response to the causative factors.

Biological Aspects

Biological research into ischemic cardiovascular disease is vast and complex; only three general aspects will be considered here. The purpose of this section is to identify where possible the relationship between coronary risk factors and the biological mechanisms of ischemic heart disease. At a general level ischemic cardiovascular disease can be thought of in terms of: (1) cellular changes in the vessel wall, atherosclerosis; (2) clot formation or thrombosis of circulating blood; and (3) the molecular interactions involved in atherosclerosis and thrombosis.

In atherosclerosis there are four important changes which take place in the vessel wall. Initially there is alteration in the integrity of the endothelial lining of the vessel. This is followed by proliferation of smooth muscle cells in the intimal layer, and synthesis and deposition by these cells of connective tissue matrix proteins. Then lipids accumulate within the proliferated smooth muscle cells and within macrophages as well as in the new connective tissue matrix. With chronic endothelial injury this process may persist so that continued lipid accumulation, smooth muscle proliferation, and calcification reduce the arterial lumen and ultimately lead to ischemia. If injury is interrupted, the process can regress and not advance beyond a stage of slight intimal thickening involving some degree of intimal smooth muscle proliferation. The initial injury to the endothelial vessel lining may result from a number of factors including hypertension, diabetes, smoking, mechanical forces, chemical agents such as lipoproteins, various toxins, immunologic injury, viruses, and other factors. One theory of atherosclerosis, the response to injury hypothesis, postulates that endothelial injury is the primary event that initiates atherosclerosis (Ross, 1981a).

Among the many functions fulfilled by endothelium is the maintenance of its own integrity. Its nonreactive surface resists thrombosis through a number of mechanisms, the synthesis of relatively large amounts of prostacyclin (PGI_2) being one such mechanism. This particular prostaglandin derivative is a potent vasodilator and antiaggregatory substance for platelets (Moncada & Vane, 1979). Another characteristic of endothelium is cell proliferation, particularly of smooth muscle cells. While the clinical sequelae of atherosclerosis depend upon the degree of proliferation, the process of cell proliferation may also be a protective mechanism. A growth factor produced by endothelial cells in culture has been identified which stimulates the synthesis of DNA and mitosis in smooth muscle cells. Growth factors from platelets and the monocyte/macrophage have also been identified in culture. The role of these growth factors in vivo is undetermined. The in vivo identification of platelet growth factor, coupled with in vivo observations that platelets adhere to injured endothelium and release their contents, suggest that platelets may play a role in smooth muscle cell migration from media to intima of the artery and proliferation in the intima. Blood monocytes are involved in the cellular changes in the vessel wall. They enter the injured intima early, phagocytosing numerous substances including lipid, and, together with smooth muscle cells, become foam cells (Gerrity, 1981; Ross, 1981a).

Coupled with these cellular changes within the vessel wall is the other intrinsic component of occlusive vascular disease, thrombosis. This takes place on the inner lining of the arterial lumen. Normally the endothelium is nonthrombogenic, keeping the vessel lining free of thrombi. However, fatty acids and various lipoproteins, particularly LDL, may interfere with the function of the endothelium so that the surface becomes damaged and is no longer nonthrombogenic. Serum lipids may therefore influence thrombogenesis through damage to the endothelium (Nordoy, 1981). Platelet function is also affected by hypercholesterolemia with an increased concentration of LDL. This increased propensity to thrombus formation has been related to changes in concentration of cholesterol and phospholipids in the platelet membrane (Shattil et al., 1977). These membrane changes are thought to have the effect of altering platelet metabolism and function, including an increased platelet sensitivity to aggregation (Carvalho, Colman, & Lees, 1974). These effects are thought not to occur with changes in serum HDL or high serum triglyceride levels (Nordoy, Strom, & Gjesdal, 1974; Nordoy et al., 1979). In experimental animals the increased thrombotic tendency associated with a high intake of saturated fat is counteracted by the addition of polyunsaturated fatty acids from both the linoleic and linolenic acid families. Human studies have made similar findings (Nordoy, 1981; Dayton et al., 1968). A series of studies has also been carried out on the effect of changes in plasma lipids on plasma coagulation and the fibrinolytic systems. No clear relationship was found, and increased coagulation with increased fibrinogen level in hyperlipoproteinemia seems to be the most consistent finding (Nordoy, 1981). The most significant link between dietary fats and thrombogenesis appears to be through the effects on the vessel wall and platelets.

SUMMARY

The anatomical focus of coronary heart disease, the arterial endothelium, is precisely defined by our knowledge of the pathology of atherosclerosis and by biological research of atherogenesis. The exact mechanisms causing the disease are only incompletely understood despite 75 years of research. Epidemiological investigation has successfully identified risk factors among which life style is overwhelmingly the most important. Nevertheless, these risk factors only partially explain the heart disease epidemic. It seems probable that there are additional aspects of our way of life yet to be researched that cause atherosclerosis. The mechanisms involved in causing the disease revolve around molecular changes related to elevated serum cholesterol and the consequent disturbance in the structure and function of the arterial wall and platelets. Many gaps in our understanding remain, particularly concerning the relationship between risk factors like a fatty diet, smoking, and physical inactivity and the biological changes of atherosclerosis.

The outstanding feature of both cancer and heart disease is that both these giant killers of the 20th century are the consequences of social and economic development and of prosperity and affluence. Since the start of industrialization and the subsequent technological revolution, people have altered their living and working environment in a way that is unprecedented. With this new environment have come new ways of living—machines do what people previously did for themselves with such efficiency that the consumption of goods and resources has become an end in itself. Industrial society no longer strives to have enough goods to sustain life; there are enough goods to sustain life, but these goods are unequally distributed. Developed society now competes with past records of production and consumption to achieve progressively greater efficiency and more and more luxury and comfort. Biologically, however, humanity has not adapted. Our diet causes cancer and heart disease, cigarettes cause cancer and heart disease, lack of activity predisposes us to heart disease, and so on. Neither have humans adapted intellectually; we cannot judge when to control the rate of social development in order to minimize its harm and optimize the good. Scientifically, humans are struggling to understand the health effects of affluence, and it is hoped this will help find ways to speed up our biological adaptation. Finally, there is the possibility that our technological ability will help us control or modify the harmful aspects of the environment and so prevent or postpone its adverse health effects. This brings us to consider the solutions to these problems. What can be done to alter the harmful health effects of western society? How effective and efficient are these strategies? In the next chapters, these are some of the issues which will be addressed.

Chapter 7

Solutions I: Reducing the Risk of Disease

In this and the two chapters following, the evidence on effective solutions to major health problems is examined. The first consideration is that of primary prevention, or methods designed to remove risk factors prior to the development of disease. Once disease occurs the effectiveness of treatment depends upon being able to change the natural history of disease. The evidence on the effectiveness of strategies and treatment in secondary and tertiary prevention (disease treatment and rehabilitation, respectively) is discussed in Chapter 8. Finally, Chapter 9 will examine the effect on health of the organization of the health care system itself.

To this point, evidence has been presented describing the health problems of society and the determinants of these problems. In the course of research, once risk factors and causes of disease have been identified, an easily made mistake is to assume that knowledge of risk is equivalent to knowledge of how to remove risk. The raison d'être of the present chapter is based on the importance of clearly distinguishing between factors which predispose to disease and knowledge of which interventions and strategies can effectively alter the risk of disease.

The studies reviewed in this chapter are organized in terms of the following risk factors: smoking, diet, alcohol consumption, driving behavior, and immune status.

METHODS

This evaluation of intervention studies requires consideration of methodological issues which have not yet been discussed. As with studies of prognosis and causation there are characteristics of the research methods employed in an intervention study that have an important bearing on the quality and therefore utility of the results. Central to the evaluation of an intervention is the concept of effectiveness. An effective maneuver is one that, when offered to an individual or group, results in the desired outcome. This depends upon two prerequisites. First, the maneuver must be capable of working under ideal circumstances; that is, it must be efficacious. Second, the recipient needs to comply with what is prescribed.

In the evaluation of either a preventive or therapeutic maneuver, the purpose of the study design is to assure that the observed outcome is truly attributable to the intervention being studied and is not due to some other factor. The other purpose is to assure that, if the intervention is effective, its effect will be measurable and not missed. The following characteristics help a study to achieve these objectives.

1. *Inclusion criteria:* The study population should be selected according to explicit inclusion criteria.
2. *Random allocation:* The allocation of subjects to the intervention must be random in order to assure comparability of treatment and control groups.
3. *Prognostic stratification:* Within a study population, at the outset of a study, the risk of developing the outcome of interest may be unequal. When this is the case, the population should be divided into subgroups of similar risk, prognostically stratified, prior to randomization.
4. *Description of maneuver:* The intervention being evaluated should be described in sufficient detail to allow it to be replicated precisely. This includes the full description of the content of the intervention, the circumstances of its administration, and by whom it is administered.
5. *Co-morbidity:* Because a second disease can influence a patient's response to a health intervention, the existence of co-morbidity (a disease additional to that being studied) should be clearly documented.
6. *Compliance:* In an efficacy trial the compliance of subjects with the intervention must be assured and evidence of this should be reported.
7. *Contamination:* It is possible for subjects in the control group to inadvertently be exposed to the intervention under study;

this is contamination. This must be guarded against and the reader told how the investigator avoided its occurrence.

8. *Co-intervention:* Subjects in the treatment or control group may be exposed unequally to therapy or interventions outside the study that affect their health. A strategy should be employed and reported which obviates this form of confounding.

9. *Diagnostic criteria:* The assessment of the outcomes of the study should follow strict criteria which can be replicated. These criteria should be reported.

10. *Comprehensive assessment of outcomes:* In the event of adverse effects resulting from an intervention, the reporting of total mortality and possibly morbidity will safeguard against these undesirable outcomes being overlooked.

11. *Complete follow-up:* All individuals entered into a trial need to be accounted for at the end. This should be identifiable in the reported results of a study.

While it is rare for all these criteria to be met in a given study each one is important to consider as their omission is a potential source of bias (Sackett, 1980).

The choice of research design for the evaluation of an intervention is limited. Nonexperimental designs such as cohort and case-control studies and the analytic survey are not appropriate for assessing the efficacy and effectiveness of interventions. An experiment, preferably with randomization is necessary in order to: (1) control adequately for the numerous potential confounding variables and (2) to permit detection of the benefits of interventions, which are often small in magnitude and are frequently limited to specific individuals and are thus easily concealed without the degree of control offered by an experiment. Many of the results discussed in this and the next chapter come from randomized controlled trials.

INTERVENTIONS TO REDUCE RISK

As with other sections it is only possible to make limited coverage of this subject and for this reason discussion will focus on major risk factors.

Reducing the Risk due to Smoking

The nonsmoking habit is undoubtedly the most direct method to reduce and ultimately eliminate the harmful effects of tobacco. However, this is not the only way. A less toxic cigarette is one alternative. It is also important to consider that only about 10% of heavy smokers die of lung cancer (MacMahon, 1981), which suggests that a factor(s) other than tobacco is benefitting the remaining 90% of smokers. There are therefore three types of intervention which will be considered: production of a safe cigarette, prevention through manipulating factors which may protect against the occurrence of harmful effects, and cessation of smoking.

A Safe Cigarette

Mortality from lung cancer in England and Wales among young men has declined by approximately 50% since 1960, despite the relatively small decline in the national consumption of tobacco. Since 1934 the tar and nicotine content and carbon monoxide yield of cigarettes in the United Kingdom have declined considerably, namely by 49%, 31%, and 11%, respectively (Wald, Doll, & Copeland, 1981). Doll (1983) reasons that these modern cigarettes are less harmful in terms of lung cancer and that this fall in mortality cannot be explained without this interpretation. The reduction in tar content of cigarettes may have played a larger part in the reduction of lung cancer in the U.K. than that with which it has been credited so far. Consistent with this hypothesis is the finding from an American study (Auerbach, Hammond, & Garfinkel, 1979) that there have been very marked reductions in the frequency of abnormal cellular changes at autopsy in the bronchial epithelium of smokers between the two periods 1955–1960 and 1970–1977. A further aspect of considerable interest concerning a safer cigarette is the relationship between the quantity of smoke inhaled and the cigarette's nicotine content.

The high dependence-producing potency of nicotine may underlie the motivation to smoke, such that a larger number of cigarettes that are low in nicotine need to be smoked to get the equivalent dose of nicotine from cigarettes with a higher nicotine content. Exposure to the tar and carbon monoxide of cigarettes could possibly be reduced by producing a cigarette low in tar and carbon monoxide but high in nicotine. The feasibility of this strategy would depend upon satisfactorily demonstrating that the increased amount of nicotine brought no added harm (Russell,

1974). Given the great difficulty in not starting to smoke, and in subsequently stopping, there is merit in a safe cigarette as a partial solution to the harm produced by cigarettes.

Control of Other Etiologic or Protective Factors

The added risk of disease from smoking varies with the types of disease and ranges from about 1.5 times for coronary heart disease to at least 10 times for lung cancer. While the number of additional cases of disease due to smoking is very large, we need to remember also that large numbers of smokers do not die prematurely. Why is this? Either there is a second harmful factor to which only a small proportion of smokers are exposed, or some protective factor is preventing the harmful effects of cigarettes in the majority of smokers. Little is known about this aspect of smoking; it may be that factors such as heredity and biological adaptation are involved. There are some relevant findings concerning the possible role of dietary vitamin A (from carrots and some other vegetables) protecting against cancer. Bjelke (1975) found that the incidence of lung cancer in smokers with a diet high in vitamin A was two-fifths of that in smokers whose diet was low in the vitamin. In this 5-year prospective study (nonexperimental) of 8,000 Norwegian men a protective effect of vitamin A was observed at each level of cigarette smoking. Similar observations have been made in a huge prospective study in Japan (Hirayama, 1979) and in some case-control studies (Basu et al., 1976; Mettlin, Graham, & Swanson, 1979). A preventive trial is needed to evaluate the practical value of vitamin A in protecting against cancer.

Cessation of Smoking

Prospective observational studies have clearly demonstrated the association of smoking with disease and of cessation of smoking in volunteers with a reduction in disease (Doll & Peto, 1976; Rogot & Murray, 1980). It would seem reasonable to infer that cessation of smoking in any smoker would be beneficial and that all smokers should be encouraged to stop smoking. However, the relationship between interventions to quit smoking and subsequent improvements in health is more complex than one is tempted to deduce from these studies. The first consideration is that individuals who give up cigarettes may have a lower risk of disease before quitting than other smokers. Certainly it seems as though individuals prone to stop smoking have characteristics that distinguish them from other smokers.

A number of characteristics have been found to be predictive of an individual's likelihood to stop smoking or to reduce the number of cigarettes smoked. The following data come from a national U.S. survey and two community surveys conducted in 1966 (Eisinger, 1972). Males were found to be more likely to stop or reduce smoking than females. Individuals acquainted with someone adversely affected by smoking were nearly three times as likely to stop smoking as other smokers. The greater number of cigarettes smoked per day, the less likely the person was to stop. The rate of stopping or reducing smoking was 44% among individuals with children under 16 years of age in the household. Cessation was more frequent among people who thought quitting was easy rather than difficult. Individuals who felt research would find cures soon for the disease caused by smoking were less likely to stop than people less optimistic of such research discoveries. From these findings it would be expected that active measures to modify smoking behavior would have variable results, depending upon the recipients of the intervention. The other variable is the intervention itself.

A basic approach to reduce exposure to cigarette smoke among smokers who are as yet unsuccessful in quitting is the set of guidelines advocated by the Royal College of Physicians (1971). These are to smoke fewer cigarettes, inhale less, smoke less of each cigarette, take fewer puffs from each cigarette, take the cigarette out of the mouth between puffs, and smoke brands with low nicotine and tar content. As discussed above, Russell (1974) considers that smokers would possibly be exposed to fewer hazards if they smoked brands high in nicotine and low in carbon monoxide and tar. Compliance with and the effectiveness of these guidelines have not been tested experimentally.

In 1964 the landmark report of the U.S. Surgeon General on smoking and health (Department of Health, Education and Welfare, 1964) was published. In the same year two new trends appeared: cigarette consumption in men started to decline and coronary heart disease mortality passed its peak and began to fall. A few months later the American Heart Association recommended a change in the American diet. The association of these events raises the possibility that these major public statements are effective interventions both in changing smoking behavior and in improving health. There is no way of knowing whether this association is cause or coincidence (Walker, 1977). Recently, however, major trials of community level interventions have been conducted.

Mass media education programs at the community level have been evaluated as a means of reducing cardiovascular risk factors, including smoking. Using three North California towns, community education alone and combined with individual counseling was successful in reducing smoking and other risk factors (Farquhar et al., 1977). The intervention was elaborate. It was designed after analysis of the knowledge deficits and media consumption patterns of the intended audience. Strategies were designed to teach specific behavioral skills, to increase motivation, to change attitudes, and to develop self-control as well as offering information. The goal was to achieve changes in smoking, exercise, and diet. The mass media campaign involved television and radio programming; weekly newspaper columns, advertisements, and stories; and bill boards, posters, and printed material posted to participants. This continued for two 9-month periods during 1973 and 1974. Counseling was offered to one high-risk subgroup in one town. This was conducted intensively over a 10-week period through group classes and home counseling sessions. The mass media program reduced cigarette consumption significantly in one town but not in the other. Individual counseling among high-risk individuals increased significantly the extent of smoking reduction beyond that achieved by community education. If an extensive mass media campaign coupled with intensive counseling can reduce smoking, what is the impact on disease incidence?

In order to test the effectiveness of smoking cessation strategies in improving health, it is preferable to study individuals rather than communities. In studies which randomize communities, control over added factors that affect health cannot be monitored adequately. For this reason, as well as difficulty identifying benefits in subgroups, those research designs with individuals as the unit of analysis rather than whole communities offer more precision (Kuller, 1980).

There are now a number of risk factor intervention trials which randomize individuals. In one trial of smoking cessation (Rose & Hamilton, 1978), which used personal interviews by the doctor as the intervention, the results were disappointing. Although smoking was significantly reduced and maintained, and symptomatology improved, there was no difference in mortality over the 7 years of the study. The results of Rose and Hamilton indicate that the benefits of stopping smoking have been overestimated by the observational studies of smoking.

In the Oslo study (Hjermann et al., 1981) the effect of a smoking and diet intervention was evaluated. The results were more encouraging. Mean tobacco consumption reduction was 45% greater in the intervention group and the incidence of myocardial infarction (fatal and nonfatal) and sudden death was 47% lower. Unfortunately, these benefits have proved difficult to reproduce.

In the Multiple Risk Factor Intervention Trial (1982) (MRFIT) 12,866 high-risk men aged 35–57 years were entered into a study of a multifactor primary prevention program. The intervention included stepped-care treatment for hypertension, counseling for cigarette smoking, and dietary advice for lowering blood cholesterol levels. Over 7 years of follow-up, risk factors diminished in both the treatment and control groups, but to a greater degree in individuals receiving the intervention. However, there was no significant difference in mortality. This may indicate that primary prevention of cardiovascular disease is ineffective, but other explanations are also feasible. The intervention in this study was most extensive; it employed group techniques, behavioral diagnosis, individual behavior techniques, and support systems (Benfari, 1981). The combination and intensity of strategies employed exceed those normally available to primary care practitioners.

With a more simple strategy (Donovan et al., 1975) antismoking advice given by the doctor at routine antenatal visits, similar results were obtained. The antismoking advice consisted of: (1) telling the patient the facts about smoking in pregnancy, (2) encouraging the patient to ask questions about these factors, (3) discussing the ways in which this could be done once the patient had agreed to try to stop smoking, and (4) following up this advice in subsequent visits, and emphasizing reinforcement, support, and maintaining contact with the patient. Some reduction in smoking was achieved. During mid-pregnancy, the treatment group had reduced its cigarette consumption to 82% of the controls' and by late pregnancy, average consumption was 9.2 cigarettes per day (56% of the controls') compared with 16.4 among controls. At birth and at 6 weeks infant weight, length, and head circumferences were similar for both groups. Maturity, placental weight, and incidence of fetal distress and perinatal mortality were also unaffected (Donovan, 1977).

The effect of stopping smoking on cancer incidence is another important question which is currently unanswered. Observational studies suggest that cessation of smoking would bring a large reduction in the frequency of cancer, as they suggest for cardiovascular disease. However, there are no randomized controlled trials of smoking cessation which specifically evaluate the modification of cancer rates (Kuller et al., 1982).

Observational studies of smoking cessation and lung function suggest that the loss in pulmonary function that has already occurred is permanent. The possible exception to this is in the minority of smokers who are susceptible to the obstructive effects of cigarette smoking. They may benefit considerably from early cessation (Kuller et al., 1982).

Discussion

Strategies to stop smoking, whether advice, counseling, behavior programs, or mass media, are of limited proven value. This is despite the highly developed nature of some of these interventions. When antismoking advice is given, in order to change smoking behavior it needs to be offered repeatedly and in a particular manner. Consideration of the characteristics of the person to whom the advice is given is also important, as some people are more prone to reduce or stop smoking than others. While these various strategies can reduce smoking their success in this regard is modest. Proscription as a preventive strategy may be a less acceptable form of behavior change than prescriptive approaches, such as smoking a safe cigarette or ingestion of a protective agent, possibly vitamin A. While the evidence concerning the effectiveness of these different strategies is often inconclusive and disappointing, it should be remembered that the reduction in tar, nicotine, and carbon monoxide yields of cigarettes may have played a greater role in the recent declines in cardiovascular disease and lung cancer than previously thought.

Changing Diet and Reducing Serum Cholesterol

The harmful effect of a cholesterol-rich diet and the subsequent regression of atheroma when the diet is discontinued have been demonstrated in animal experiments (Chapter 6). In the large observational studies comparing diet in different countries, the correlation of diet to serum cholesterol and coronary disease mortality is also moderately well documented (Chapter 6). The principal dietary components incriminated are saturated fatty acids. To a lesser extent, daily caloric intake, essential fatty acids, dietary fiber, alcohol, and salt also contribute to the observed deleterious effects of the modern diet. However, from studies within the same cultural group or of individuals there is no sound correlation between diet and coronary heart disease (Oliver, 1981). In the case of cancer, in a very large prospective study in Japan a moderately high correlation between low green-yellow vegetable intake (an important source of vitamin A) and cancer incidence has been observed (Hirayama, 1979). Dietary intervention studies in humans have not found a change in diet as effective in improving health as expected.

Interventions designed to change diet that have been evaluated in terms of reduction in serum cholesterol have been found moderately successful. The mass media campaign employed in the Stanford Heart Disease Prevention Program (Farquhar et al., 1977) reduced dietary saturated fat intake by well over 20 g/day in both the general population sample and high-risk individuals. Reductions in serum cholesterol were significant in both groups, but were greater in high-risk subjects. Face-to-face instruction brought no added benefit beyond that achieved by the media campaign, whereas individual instruction was effective with smoking reduction. At the national level, U.S. dietary habits have changed significantly since the American Heart Association recommended a change in the American diet in 1964. Between 1963 and 1975 there was a 57% reduction in per capita consumption of animal fats and oils and a 44% increase in vegetable oils and fats. Per capita consumption of milk, cream, butter, and eggs has also declined. The roles these dietary changes have played in the decline of coronary disease mortality since then can only be speculated (Walker, 1977). A small number of dietary and drug trials have endeavored to test this relationship; their limited success has been diminished by some disconcerting harmful effects.

The dietary and cholesterol-lowering interventions in the major primary prevention trials on individuals have been limited to cardiovascular disease prevention. There have been no dietary trials of cancer prevention. Surprisingly, a low saturated fat diet has not been evaluated. The dietary interventions have prescribed the substitution of saturated fat with polyunsaturated fat, such as in the Los Angeles Veterans Administration Trial (Dayton et al., 1968), the Helsinki Mental Hospital Study (Miettinen et al., 1972), and the Anti-Coronary Club Trial (Rinzler, 1968). Similar diets were prescribed in the multiple factor intervention trials (Hjermann et al., 1981; MRMIT, 1982). The primary prevention drug trials have employed cholesterol-lowering agents: clofibrate in both the WHO Cooperative Trial (Committee of Principal Investigators,

1978) and the United Airlines Trial, and cholestyramine in the Lipid Research Clinics Coronary Primary Prevention Trial (1984).

The Los Angeles Veterans Administration Trial (Dayton et al., 1968) was the first to be completed. The trial studied 846 men with a mean age of 66 years. Half were randomized to a conventional diet and half to an experimental diet. The conventional diet contained 40% fat calories, mostly of animal origin. Two thirds of these calories were provided by vegetable oils in the experimental diet, with total fat calories maintained at approximately 40%. The primary outcome was new coronary events. It is important to note that, due to the age of the study population, a proportion already had clinical features of coronary heart disease at the start of the study. The results showed the mean difference in serum cholesterol to be 13% lower in the experimental group. There was no significant difference in coronary disease incidence but a favorable trend existed for nonfatal myocardial infarction. There was a statistically significant increase in nonatherosclerotic deaths in the experimental group as well as an increased incidence of gallstones.

The Helsinki Mental Hospital Study (Miettinen et al., 1972) was nonrandomized and had a number of methodological weaknesses (Oliver, 1980). Potential confounding variables were not controlled optimally, the study population changed during the study, and the endpoints were not defined clearly. A polyunsaturated fat diet was given to the experimental group. The results showed a 15% reduction of raised serum cholesterol and a significant reduction in coronary disease, but deaths definitely due to coronary heart disease showed no significant difference. An observed excess of noncardiovascular deaths in the experimental group was not statistically significant. In the Anti-Coronary Club Trial (Rinzler, 1968) the results suggested that a prudent diet reduced coronary disease, but the poor design precludes placing confidence in the findings. On the basis of these diet trials the effectiveness of substituting polyunsaturated vegetable oils for animal fats in reducing the incidence of heart disease is inconclusive.

The single-risk-factor drug trials have investigated the hypothesis that reduction in serum cholesterol will result in a lower incidence of coronary heart disease. The WHO Cooperative Trial (Committee of Principal Investigators, 1978) was a very well designed and executed randomized double blind controlled trial of clofibrate. The study comprised 15,745 healthy men aged 30–59 years. Serum cholesterol was reduced by 9% in the treatment group. This was coupled with a similarly modest but statistically significant reduction in nonfatal myocardial infarcts. The frequency of fatal heart attacks was similar in control and experimental groups. The very disconcerting finding was a 25% excess of deaths from all causes in the clofibrate group. There was also a significant excess of cholecystectomies due to gallstones in the experimental group. The United Airlines Trial also evaluated clofibrate. However, this study was not randomized, comparability of study and control groups was not established, and numerous biases were probable. Therefore, the results are of little value (Oliver, 1980).

The most significant investigation into cholesterol reduction and the incidence of coronary heart disease is the Lipid Research Clinics Trial (1984). This study investigated the efficacy of cholestyramine (an anion exchange resin) among asymptomatic men aged 35–59 years with primary hypercholesterolemia. All men entered into the study had plasma cholesterol levels of 265 mg/dl or greater and low-density-lipoprotein cholesterol (LDL-C) levels of 190 mg/dl or greater. While participants were free of coronary heart disease they were all at high risk. They were randomized to receive either cholestyramine or a placebo for an average of 7.4 years. Both groups followed a moderate cholesterol-lowering diet. The study group experienced reductions in total serum cholesterol and LDL-C that were, respectively, 8.5% and 12.6% greater than occurred in the placebo group. Coronary disease deaths and nonfatal heart attacks were reduced by 24% and 19%, respectively, in the cholestyramine group. In addition, in the treatment group the incidence of new positive exercise tests, angina, and coronary by-pass surgery was reduced by 25%, 20%, and 21%, respectively. Violent and accidental deaths were greater in the treatment group, so that the risk of death from all causes was only slightly and not significantly reduced. A significant increase in gallstones or cholecystectomies was not observed, in contrast to the diet and clofibrate trials.

Discussion

Obtaining experimental evidence to support the internationally observed diet–cholesterol–heart disease relationship has been slow and difficult. For the general population the impact on heart disease of dietary changes such as reduction of saturated fat, increasing P/S ratio (the ratio of polyunsaturated to saturated fat), and reduction in total fat calories has not been demonstrated.

While the benefits of such changes for middle-aged men with elevated serum cholesterol are not fully investigated, they are understood much better than previously.

Reductions in serum cholesterol ranging from 9% to 15% have been obtained repeatedly with nonharmful strategies. The interventions that have demonstrated effectiveness are institutional low cholesterol diets, mass media campaigns, prescription and monitoring of a low cholesterol diet, and cholestyramine. In the Lipid Research Clinics Trial (1984), the diet protocol was complied with effectively over 7 years. The diet included reduction in total calories, cholesterol, total fat, saturated fat, and an increase in the P/S ratio.

However, the evidence that a dietary intervention alters the incidence of heart disease is inconclusive. The well-designed Veterans Administration Trial (Dayton et al., 1968) showed no effect and only the nonrandomized Helsinki study (Miettinen et al., 1972) demonstrated a reduction in coronary disease incidence.

Cholestyramine-induced reduction in serum cholesterol in men with hypercholesterolemia has produced the most substantial and definite reductions in coronary heart disease observed to the present. Significant reductions in morbidity, nonfatal heart attacks, and coronary deaths have all been demonstrated. These benefits have been attributed to the reduction in serum LDL-C levels.

Multiple Risk Factor Reduction

Rather than testing interventions for single risk factors some trials have been conducted to reduce multiple risk factors. The major studies of this type conducted on individuals are the Oslo study and the MRFIT.

The Oslo Study (Hjermann et al., 1981) investigated the impact of dietary and antismoking advice on the incidence of coronary heart disease in high-risk men aged 40–49 years. The study population comprised 1,232 healthy normotensive (systolic blood pressure below 150 mm Hg) men, all of whom had a serum cholesterol of 290–380 mg/dl and of whom 80% smoked. They were randomized either to receive the intervention or to the control group. The intervention included an individual talk on risk factors, individualized dietary advice from a dietitian, antismoking advice given individually, an information session for wives, and an inquiry every 6 months into smoking and eating habits at the time of scheduled reexaminations by a physician. Diet changed significantly in the study group and smoking declined modestly. Serum cholesterol declined to approximately 13% lower than that of the control group. At the end of the study, fatal and nonfatal myocardial infarction and sudden death were 47% lower in the intervention group compared with controls. In analyzing the data, the reduction in disease incidence correlated with the reduction in serum cholesterol and to a lesser extent with smoking reduction.

The Multiple Risk Factor Intervention Trial (1982) assessed interventions to reduce three major risk factors: elevated blood pressure, elevated serum cholesterol, and smoking. Middle-aged men with no clinical evidence of coronary heart disease but who were in the upper 10% of a risk scale based on smoking, serum cholesterol, and blood pressure were entered into the study. Of these men 6,428 were randomly assigned to receive the intervention; nearly the same number received no intervention and were assigned to continue with their usual sources of health care in the community. The controls were invited to return once a year for a medical assessment.

The initial phase of the intervention was an intensive integrated effort to lower the three major risk factors by means of individual counseling and 10 weekly group discussions. Following this, individual counseling was planned and executed by an intervention team of health professionals. The men receiving the intervention were seen every 4 months and more often as needed for intervention purposes. Hypertension was treated with weight reduction, stepped drug therapy, and mild sodium restriction. The dietary intervention sought to encourage the development of lifelong shopping, cooking, and eating patterns rather than to prescribe a specific diet. Individual nutritional goals were set to lower serum cholesterol by an amount determined by the serum level at the time of entry. Eating patterns were recommended that reduced saturated fat intake to less than 10% of calories (later reduced to 8%) and dietary cholesterol intake to less than 300 mg/day (later reduced to 250 mg/day), and increased polyunsaturated fat intake to 10% of calories. Smokers were urged to quit. Dosage reduction was recommended only as a step towards cessation. Conventional behavior modification techniques were used throughout the trial. The 10 weekly group sessions and 5-day quit clinics during the final years are reported as having been particularly successful (Benfari, 1981).

Risk factor reduction for the intervention group was significantly greater than for controls for all three factors at each annual visit.

The average reduction in blood pressure, 6 years into the trial, was 10.5 mmHg in the intervention group and 7.3 mmHg in the controls. Smoking quit rates (thiocyante adjusted) at 12 months were 31% for the study group and 12% for controls, and at 6 years, these proportions had increased to 46% and 20%, respectively. Reductions in serum cholesterol were less in the study group and greater than anticipated in the controls. At 12 months, the reductions were 10.4 mg/dl in the intervention group and 3.4 mg/dl among controls, and by 6 years, these reductions were 12.1 mg/dl and 7.5 mg/dl, respectively. These changes were principally in LDL-C and not HDL-C (MRFIT, 1982).

Surprisingly, however, mortality from coronary heart disease was 17.9 deaths per 1,000 in the intervention group and 19.3 per 1,000 among controls. This difference of 7.1% between the two groups is not statistically significant. Mortality from all causes was 41.2 deaths/1,000 and 40.4/1,000 in the treatment and control groups, respectively. Several explanations for these findings are possible. The interventions may not be effective. Alternatively they may be beneficial, but this was not demonstrated in this study because the death rate among controls was lower than expected and the reduction in risk factors in men not receiving the intervention was greater than anticipated. Third, a trend was observed in the data suggesting that men without hypertension benefited from the intervention, whereas there was no apparent difference between study group and controls for the subgroup with hypertension. A possible explanation is that the relatively adverse response of the hypertensive subgroup has concealed the benefit to the others (MRFIT, 1982).

Discussion

When each study is considered separately, it is easy to be pessimistic about risk factor intervention. This view may not be justified. On the positive side there are a number of major findings and trends which are consistent with risk factor change being both possible and beneficial. Death rates from heart disease, stroke, and lung cancer (men 30–49 years) are falling. The consumption of fatty foods is changing favorably. Tobacco consumption is declining and the tar and nicotine content of cigarettes is being reduced. The associations of a fatty diet with heart disease, and smoking with heart and lung disease, are indisputable. A change in diet can consistently reduce serum cholesterol, and now it has been shown that an intervention (cholestyramine) that reduces serum cholesterol decreases the incidence of coronary heart disease. The Oslo trial (Hjermann et al., 1981) brought much of this evidence together by demonstrating that dietary and antismoking advice in normotensive men led to a fall in coronary heart disease. All this evidence indicates not only that dietary change and smoking reduction are beneficial, but that there is a general societal change involving improvement in diet and smoking behavior, and a concurrent reduction in vascular disease and some cancer.

When these changes in behavior and disease incidence occur in the control group of a risk factor trial, it becomes increasingly difficult to demonstrate the benefits of the intervention. General societal changes in diet and smoking may have been the co-interventions responsible for the unexpected improvements in serum cholesterol and smoking in the control group of the Multiple Risk Factor Intervention Trial. Therefore, if such a trial had been conducted before 1964, when changes in behavior and disease rates started to appear, the results may have been different.

The negative results of some trials of smoking and diet and of the Multiple Risk Factor Intervention Trial (1982) may also have been affected by a further factor. Despite the general benefit of a low fat diet and stopping smoking, most probably this benefit is not shared equally by everyone. For example, the elderly men in the Los Angeles Veterans Administration trial (Dayton et al., 1968) may not have been as responsive to dietary improvements as younger men. Similarly, there is a suggestion in the MRFIT that the hypertensive men did not experience the possibly beneficial response of those who were normotensive. There are therefore plausible reasons to support an optimistic view towards changing cardiovascular risk factors despite the mixed nature of present evidence.

Reducing the Consumption of Alcohol

Most of the major risk factors relevant to health in the 20th century are peculiar to this century. By contrast, the consumption of alcohol dates back to ancient times and forms an intrinsic component of much human society.

The biological toxicity of alcohol and the association of various health problems with its consumption are well established (Smith, 1981b). Of less certainty is how consumption and damage are related, what determines consumption, and, particularly, how the damage can be avoided. Prevention through universal restrictions is not acceptable to western society, as demonstrated by the history of prohibition. More subtle strategies are needed.

Interventions to curb the intake of alcohol have not been evaluated by controlled trials as has been done with smoking and diet. Consequently, our understanding of ways to change drinking behavior is based on observational data only.

Health education, as a method of changing behavior, has the advantage of being acceptable to the public whereas regulatory methods such as price control are generally unpopular. Public health education campaigns about alcohol can make some change in attitudes toward drink and drunkenness but have not been shown to be effective in reducing consumption (Plant, Pirie, Kreitman, 1979). In order to be successful, behavior change strategies need to be based on an individual's attitudes, motivation, and sources of reinforcement (Marshall, 1980). For these reasons, it is logical (but not necessarily effective) to complement mass media campaigns with individual health education provided by medical practitioners, nurses, other health workers, or teachers. The effectiveness of individual health education in changing alcohol consumption or problems due to alcohol has not been demonstrated (Edwards et al., 1977; Smith, 1981c).

The other method to influence drinking is by regulation of price, alcohol availability, and advertising. More positive evidence exists concerning these strategies than for health education, but again the data are only from uncontrolled observational studies. The most consistent findings relate price to both consumption and damage due to alcohol. The relative price of alcohol is inversely related to consumption, so that as price falls people drink more. This has been observed in many countries. Deaths are also affected. The death rate from liver cirrhosis increases as the relative price of alcohol declines (Smith, 1981b). One of the clearest illustrations of this relationship comes from the estimates of alcohol consumption, relative price, and cirrhosis deaths in Ontario from 1928 to 1967 (Table 7.1) (Popham, Schmidt, & de Lint, 1975). From these data it is tempting to conclude that a deliberate increase in the price of alcohol would result in changes in consumption and deaths; however, this assumption has not been tested (Smith, 1981c).

The relationship between availability of alcohol and consumption is not as consistent as for price. There are cases where the relaxation of licensing laws has resulted in increased consumption, but this is not universal (Smith, 1981b; Wilson, 1980). The situation

TABLE 7.1: Consumption of alcohol, relative price of alcohol, and deaths from liver cirrhosis, Ontario, 1928–1967

Year	Per capita alcohol consumption in liters of absolute alcohol	Relative price	Deaths from liver cirrhosis per 100,000 population
1928	2.81	0.102	4.4
1931	2.64	0.112	4.0
1934	2.09	0.137	4.2
1937	3.36	0.086	4.5
1940	3.64	0.074	5.0
1943	4.91	0.064	4.8
1946	5.82	0.069	5.4
1949	7.18	0.058	7.2
1952	7.32	0.051	7.7
1955	7.55	0.047	8.8
1958	7.96	0.043	11.0
1961	8.14	0.043	11.6
1964	8.73	0.039	11.9
1967	8.91	0.035	13.2

Source: R.E. Popham, W. Schmidt, and L. de Lint, 1975. The prevention of alcoholism: Epidemiological studies of the effects of government control measures. British Journal of Addiction 70:131. Reproduced by permission from the British Journal of Addiction and the authors.

concerning advertising is also unclear. When British Columbia introduced a total ban on alcohol advertising in 1976, there were no marked changes in alcohol consumption (Moser, 1979). Important to note is that media from the United States and other Canadian provinces continued to be received, so the effect of this regulation cannot be evaluated with confidence.

On the basis of available evidence the only measures that appear to influence alcohol consumption are governmental regulations and particularly the liquor taxes which determine the relative price of alcohol. The other approach to the problems due to alcohol is to direct interventions at reducing the damage caused by alcohol. This is the basis of legislation concerning drinking and driving.

Promoting Safe Driving Behavior

Quantitatively, deaths due to accidents are second only to heart disease and cancer, but more potential years of life are lost due to accidents than to any other cause. Motor vehicle mortality accounts for more than half of all accidental deaths, and driver behavior is responsible in the vast majority of cases. The problem is therefore one of finding ways of promoting safe driving behavior.

Driver Education

A direct and logical strategy to improve the safety of driving would seem to be driver education. However, driving training for young teenagers can have an adverse general effect in addition to any change which may occur in individual driver competence. Early studies showed accident rates to be lower in drivers with driver education than among other drivers (Allgaier, 1964). American high school students who opt for driver classes differ from other students in tending to have a higher intelligence and to be less aggressive and less impulsive (Conger, Miller, & Rainey, 1966). Observations of accident rates in drivers with driver training and in those without need to control for these differences in order to assess the true effect of driver education.

A most important effect of driver education is that it increases the number of new drivers on the road (Shaoul, 1975). In an American study of driver education (Robertson & Zador, 1978) in 27 states the teenage death rate from motor vehicle accidents was related to the proportion of teenagers who received high school driver education. Through driver education, students aged 16–17 years obtained a driving license that they otherwise would not get until 18 years of age or older. Fatal crash involvement among licensed drivers was unaltered by the education programs, and the number of road deaths among 16-year-olds was much higher due to the increased number of drivers of this age. It is estimated that at least 2,000 deaths of Americans under 18 years would have been avoided in 1975 had driver education not existed. This study and an English study (Shaoul, 1975) with similar findings indicate the importance of evaluation of educational programs that have the net effect of increasing exposure to the risk of a road accident.

Mass Media and Seat Belt Usage

Seat belt usage is an effective measure in the reduction of road accident deaths. Despite availability, seat belt usage is often low. A number of evaluations of mass media campaigns to promote the use of seat belts have been conducted. None have shown a beneficial effect. In order to overcome the methodological weaknesses of these studies, Robertson et al. (1974) employed a dual television cable used for marketing studies to promote seat belt use. The dual cable system served 13,800 households, with each household receiving only one of the two cables. High quality messages designed to promote seat belt use appeared for 9 months on one cable. The recipients of the other cable served as the control group. Seat belt use in the community was monitored by road checks for 1 month prior to and for the 9 months of the television showing. Car license plates allowed linkage to addresses and thus to the particular cable. No differences in seat belt usage was observed. From these studies, mass media alone does not appear to be effective in promoting the use of seat belts.

Legislation

Legislation, in comparison with education and mass media campaigns, has been found to change both driving behavior and road accident mortality and morbidity. Legislation concerning seat belt usage and drinking and driving serve as illustrations.

The legislation for compulsory seat belt wearing was first introduced in the state of Victoria, Australia in December 1970. Soon afterward the other states and New Zealand followed suit, making Australia and New Zealand the first countries in the world with such legislation. A penalty of $20.00 for noncompliance was introduced. During the preceding decade in Victoria, road accident deaths steadily rose to 1,061 in 1970. After the introduction of compulsory seat belt wearing, this number fell to 900/year and remained at this level until 1974 (Trinca & Dooley, 1975). A similar decline occurred in the other states. In New South Wales car occupant deaths declined from 860 in 1971 to 701 in 1972 (Henderson & Wood, 1973). Concurrently death rates among pedestrians, pedal, and motor cyclists continued to increase. The legislation did not apply to children under 8 years of age among whom the injury and mortality pattern was unchanged (Trinca & Dooley, 1975).

The greatest protection from seat belt usage was noted in car occupants involved in frontal-impact collisions. A very large decrease in severe head and facial injuries occurred; the frequency of these injuries was 23% with seat belts compared with 79% without seat belts among patients admitted to hospital following frontal-impact collisions (Trinca & Dooley, 1975). Spinal injuries were reduced (Burke, 1973); chest injuries did not appear to be affected significantly. Little added protection was afforded to individuals in side-impact collisions although head injuries were less common. Seat belts themselves caused some injury but these were most probably far less serious than the injuries the belt prevents. Ten percent of car occupants admitted to hospital after frontal-impact collisions showed injuries directly attributable to the wearing of seat belts (Trinca & Dooley, 1975).

These results indicate that the effect of seat belt legislation varies with the type of collision as well as adding a small amount of injury due to the belt itself in some accidents. Overall, however, the net effect of the legislation has been a significant reduction in road accident mortality and morbidity associated with a large proportion of car occupants wearing seat belts. Other factors which could have explained the observed decline in injuries do not appear to have been in effect. Random surveys during the daytime showed seat belt usage following the legislation in Victoria to be 85%, while a smaller percentage of car occupants in crashes were found to be wearing their belt. In 1973, 50% of drivers and 33% of front seat passengers injured in accidents were wearing their belt at the time of the accident (Henderson & Wood, 1973; Trinca & Dooley, 1975). Following the Australian and New Zealand experience, other countries followed suit with similar seat belt legislation.

The other major focus of road safety legislation is the prevention of driving while under the influence of alcohol. Reductions in road accident mortality in Victoria during the early 1970s following seat belt legislation were further reduced during the remainder of the decade by a package of interventions designed primarily to curb drinking and driving. Despite the substantial increases in both population and cars, the road toll in Victoria declined from 1,061 in 1970 to 657 in 1980 (Joint Standing Committee on Road Safety, 1982).

The Victorian package of measures included intensified random breath testing for alcohol, increased penalties for drunk driving, and several major publicity campaigns. During the period between the initial introduction of random breath testing in July 1976 and late 1978, the road toll did not fall significantly. The enforcement of the law was at a low level until October 1978. At that time, a program of periods of intensified enforcement was started, supported by mass media publicity that stressed both the risks of being caught for drunk driving and the associated severe penalties. In December 1978 the penalties doubled. A dramatic fall in mortality and blood alcohol concentration of drivers followed (McDermott & Hughes, 1982). These benefits have been maintained in contrast to the waning phenomenon observed in other countries (Ross, 1981b).

Discussion

Driving behavior is an outstanding example of significant changes having been induced successfully through legislation. Seat belt legislation and random breath testing (RBT) legislation, when accompanied by adequate law enforcement, penalties, and publicity (of RBT), can effectively reduce road accident mortality and morbidity. This dramatic preventive potential places road safety legislation as one of the major primary preventive measures introduced this century. By contrast, driver education can increase road deaths by increasing the number of young drivers on the road; media publicity in isolation is probably ineffective in changing driver behavior.

Immunization

To this point, all the interventions discussed have related to the primary prevention of chronic diseases and accidents. The importance of these interventions is derived principally from the magnitude of the health problems they are designed to prevent rather than from their modest effectiveness. Difficulty in developing effective strategies to change unhealthy and hazardous behavior is a major problem for preventive medicine. Present knowledge of efficacious methods to promote a healthy life style is in its infancy; this is similar to the stage in the history of vaccination reached in the 18th century, when variolation preceded the introduction of smallpox vaccination. Nearly two centuries later immunization stands out as the single most important and effective medical measure in the prevention of disease. The success of immunization is manifested by the absence of diseases such as smallpox, tetanus, diphtheria, polio, and others.

Diphtheria and tetanus vaccines provide almost perfect immunization. Three injections in infancy followed by one booster of inactivated toxins resulted in almost lifelong immunity. The remarkable effectiveness of tetanus toxoid immunization is illustrated by the rarity of tetanus in war injuries among vaccinated soldiers. In American servicemen in World War II there was less than 1 case per 200,000 injuries (Edsall, 1959). Diphtheria immunization has its major effect on preventing symptomatic disease but does not stop individuals carrying the organism or spreading the infection (Miller et al., 1972).

Whooping cough (pertussis) vaccine, by contrast, provides only partial protection from disease. The vaccine is a relatively crude preparation and contains the majority of the organism's constituents. The antigenic component of the organism has not yet been isolated. In the Medical Research Council trials (1959) it was shown that from among the 19 whooping cough vaccines evaluated it was possible to produce a substantial reduction in the attack rate among contacts. In those cases where vaccination failed to give complete protection, vaccination reduced the severity and duration of the disease.

The first polio vaccine (Salk) was evaluated in the early 1950's and was found to be 80–90% effective against paralytic poliomyelitis (Salk and Salk, 1978). The introduction of the Salk vaccine in the mid-1950's and later of the oral Sabin vaccine have resulted in a dramatic decline in polio to the point where its occurrence is now extremely rare. Today the more commonly used vaccine is the trivalent oral polio vaccine (TOPV), which is a live attenuated vaccine with an effectiveness of 90% against all three strains of polio virus (Young, 1979b).

A live attenuated measles vaccine was developed in 1958. In the original large scale trial of the vaccine protection was provided against the disease in at least 84% of immunized children (Medical Research Council, 1977). In subsequent surveys, a wide range in serological response to vaccination has been observed: 29–94%, depending upon the age at the time of vaccination (Christopher et al., 1983). The advantage of a higher rate of effective immunity with vaccination at 15 months of age over that induced by vaccination at 12 months needs to be balanced with the need for protection between 12 and 15 months given the significant risk of measles at this age. Immunity from vaccination does not wane over 15 years and possibly is lifelong. Compulsory measles vaccination in the United States has resulted in a dramatic decline in incidence; whereas measles is a significant problem in Australia, where vaccination is not compulsory. In 1981 there were 2,200 hospital admissions for measles and five deaths in the state of New South Wales (population: 5 million). Efficacy is not perfect and vaccine failure does occur. In a recent survey in Australia 17% of measles cases occurred in immunized children. The clinical presentation of measles in vaccinated individuals has been described as measles without the rash and is characterized by malaise, sore eyes, and a running nose (Christopher et al., 1983).

An effective mumps vaccine with a live attentuated virus has been available since 1966. A single subcutaneous inoculation produces protective levels of antibodies in more than 95% of cases (Baum & Litman, 1979). This should be given at 1 year of age or at 15 months with other vaccines.

In the case of rubella, vaccination is given to protect against the congenital rubella syndrome. Surveys show that 75% of adults are immune to rubella. The live attenuated virus boosts the immunity acquired through infection and provides immunity for those lacking natural protection (Trinca, 1979).

One of the greatest successes of vaccination and primary prevention has been the eradication of smallpox. In 1967 the World Health Organization launched a global campaign against variola major. At that time smallpox was endemic in more than 30 countries. The success of the program is attributable to several factors, including the development and availability of stable freeze-dried vaccines, advanced techniques of vaccination, greatly upgraded case identification and reporting, and the technique of surveillance containment. Since October 1975 there has not been a reported case of smallpox in the world (Henderson, 1976).

In summary, vaccination is most important both in maintaining and improving public health. In addition to the above types of immunization, many other vaccines are in use, description of which is beyond present purposes. New vaccines continue to be developed, such as the recently evaluated hepatitis B vaccine (Szmuness et al., 1980). Research into immunization is now branching out from the prevention of bacterial and viral infections into antitumour vaccines and vaccination against parasitic infections. The current status of primary prevention is therefore based on predominantly biological interventions. By comparison, behavioral interventions are in an early stage of development.

SUMMARY

Reducing the risk of disease is complex and difficult, and success has been variable. With infectious disease the effectiveness of immunization has approached perfection, but efforts to reduce heart disease and cancer by changing diet and smoking have been disappointing and confusing. Moderate success has been achieved in finding methods to reduce road injuries.

Educational strategies in primary prevention are generally of limited effectiveness. Although education, advice, and behavior modification techniques can alter dietary and smoking behavior, these changes have not reduced disease incidence or mortality. The risk of road accident injury in the population can be increased by teenage driver education programs; mass media messages do not change driving behavior. The media is effective, however, against drunk driving when employed as a component of a legislative package designed to reduce drinking and driving.

Legislation is effective in a number of areas of prevention. Alcohol consumption and cirrhosis deaths, road accident injury and mortality, tar and nicotine content in cigarettes, and compliance with vaccinations are all benefited by appropriate legislation. Particularly effective is road safety legislation when it is part of a package comprising media messages, effective law enforcement, and significant penalties.

Surprising and disappointing results have been found in the evaluation of interventions involving multiple risk factors. Contrary to our understanding of the multifactorial etiology of coronary heart disease prevention through multiple risk factor intervention has not proved effective. In fact, the most successful strategy to prevent coronary heart disease in a high-risk population is a highly specific single factor, cholestyramine. Medication in the form of cholestyramine is the most effective and safe known method to reduce blood cholesterol and coronary heart disease. Until such time as effective measures to alter life style are shown to reduce heart disease and cancer the major primary prevention measures of today remain vaccinations and legislation. The primary prevention of infectious disease through immunization has been the most successful of all preventive measures in this century, and vaccination continues to be the principal means for maintaining control over a large number of infectious diseases.

Chapter 8

Solutions II: The Search for Effective Therapy

Although health depends upon a multitude of factors, many of which are unrelated to medical therapy, society relies heavily on medical technology and the treatment of disease to protect its health. Medical care is given a central role in western society as a major determinant of health.

Disease is the outcome of a long process of interaction between a number of factors. The combined effect of heredity, behavior, and environment results in disease for some of the population, while the majority live to old age relatively free of sickness. Despite the fact that disease has its origin in events and circumstances that precede the onset of symptoms, most resources are focused on disease rather than on its determinants. Part of this disease orientation is the belief that medicine is all-powerful and can be relied upon to halt the progression of disease and save the lives of those afflicted.

Recently the sanctity of medicine has been challenged, from which a debate has developed (Illich, 1975). The question is, how much is health or illness attributable to medical therapy? On one side are the proponents for medicine, who draw upon the advances of medical science to support their argument (Beeson, 1980; McDermott, 1978; Thomas, 1978). On the one side are those who seek direct epidemiological and experimental evidence before crediting medical care with these achievements (Cochrane, 1972). The latter are exemplified by the work of McKeown (1979), in which changes in environment and behavior are placed ahead of medical therapy as determinants of health. McKeown's analysis has been described in detail previously (Chapter 4).

Beeson (1980), in a review of changes in medical therapy, has identified an imposing list of medical advances achieved during much of this century. He shows that the recommended use of ineffective measures has fallen markedly, while a greatly increased proportion of currently accepted treatment is considered to be effective. Of these changes pharmacotherapy has seen remarkable growth, with developments in antimicrobial agents, synthetic adrenal steroids, and other hormonal preparations including insulin, anticonvulsants, diuretics, immunosuppressives, and psychotropic drugs. The morbidity of schizophrenia and Parkinson's disease have been reduced dramatically through phenothiazines and levodopa, respectively. In surgery many disorders and injuries can now be treated effectively, where previously little could be done. Successful surgical treatment has been developed for valvular and congenital heart disease. Similarly, great advances have occurred in the operative management of joint disease, coronary heart disease, and genitourinary disorders. Medically, problems of fluid and electrolyte balance, renal failure, respiratory disease, cardiac arrhythmias, skin disorders, leukemia, erythroblastosis due to Rh incompatibility, and many other hematological problems are effectively treatable today. A diversity of cardiovascular and gastrointenstinal disorders for which therapy used to be ineffective can now be treated successfully. The advances in the prevention and treatment of infective disease with vaccines and antibiotics, respectively, have been outstanding in their own right, but the control of infections has also allowed many other achievements to occur, particularly in cardiothoracic and orthopedic surgery. Such evidence cannot be ignored. It is indisputable that medical science has improved the health of many individuals, as any hemophiliac, insulin-dependent diabetic, or epileptic would affirm.

In addition to the unquestionable benefits of medicine, many treatments have proved to be ineffective, harmful, or excessively costly. For certain heart attack patients, treatment in a coronary care unit has been shown to be no more effective than home care (Hill, Hampton, & Mitchell, 1978). Prolonged bed rest following a heart attack used to be universally accepted treatment, until early ambulation appeared to be no less effective (Levine & Lown, 1951). Findings such as these demonstrate the value of testing the effectiveness of new therapies before they are put into general use. This has led to a scientific skepticism which in its most orthodox form accepts no new measures unless proved by rigorous randomized double blind controlled experiments. This new attitude has drawn attention to the vast amount of current medical treatment that has been inadequately evaluated. In fact, in the majority of accepted medical therapies effectiveness is based on clinical observations and biological reasoning rather than on the findings of strict experimental assessment. When biomedically sound treatment is assessed under rigorously controlled conditions, therapeutic benefits have proved difficult to identify, as in the case of coronary care units.

The purpose of this chapter is to illustrate the importance of evaluating new medical interventions and to seek randomized controlled trial evidence wherever possible. As Cochrane (1972) points out, the credit for this experimental approach to clinical medicine should go to Sir Austin Bradford Hill. First, the investigation of several major interventions will be discussed, followed by a description of some of the methodological issues pertinent to the process of identifying effective methods of disease management.

THE SEARCH FOR EFFECTIVE THERAPY

During the last 25 years declines in mortality have been observed in heart disease and stroke, as well as in some cancers. Such changes can result from either a decline in incidence or reduced severity of disease. Of concern to medical science is the fact that there is little direct controlled evidence to suggest that medical treatment has effected a decrease in severity of the major chronic diseases. This is surprising given the great advances in medical science, and particularly as the principal function of treatment is to halt progression or reduce severity of disease. In this section the search for effective therapy for some selected cancers and some forms of vascular disease will be discussed.

Cancer

Breast cancer is the most common cancer in women. A number of trials of different forms of treatment involving surgery, radiotherapy, and chemotherapy have been conducted, but none, with the possible exception of surgery with adjuvant chemotherapy (Lacour et al., 1984), have been shown to be clearly superior. The significant predictor of survival is the stage of the disease at the time of diagnosis. Early detection therefore offers a possible hope of improving the effectiveness of treatment.

The hypothesis that screening for presymptomatic breast cancer would improve survival is well supported by observational studies of the natural history of breast cancer (Kelsey, 1979). The first randomized trial of breast screening was that of the Health Insurance Plan of New York (Shapiro, 1977). This trial was designed to evaluate the effect of periodic screening with clinical examination and mammography on breast cancer mortality among women aged 40 to 64 years. The study involved about 62,000 women, 31,000 in the treatment group and 31,000 controls. The women in the treatment group were offered screening examinations; 65% attended the initial examination and were offered three additional examinations at annual intervals unless earlier follow-up or biopsy was indicated. The majority of this group (88%) had at least one additional annual examination. Screening consisted of a clinical examination; mammography involving two views of each breast; and an interview to obtain relevant demographic information and a health history. Control women continued to receive their usual medical care. Mammography and clinical examination contributed independently to the detection of breast cancer. For women under 50 years of age, clinical examination alone detected 61% of breast cancers, and 19% were detected by mammography alone. Among women 50 years and older, the numbers of cancers detected by the two modalities separately were similar. Mortality from causes other than breast cancer was similar in the screened and unscreened groups, but breast cancer mortality was lower among those screened, being two thirds of the unscreened group. This benefit was not observed in women under 50 years of age. Similar findings have been reported in subsequent trials of breast screening (Miller & Bulbrook, 1982). These are important findings given that breast cancer mortality has not been falling, and medical and surgical treatment probably do little to change the death rate.

The effect of cervical screening, by contrast, has not been evaluated directly. Consequently, it is not possible to estimate the proportion of the decline in cancer of the cervix which may or may not be attributable to screening. The fall in cervical cancer mortality started before screening was introduced, and this plus the absence of randomized trial evidence have fueled debate over the value of screening and have made the interpretation of the available evidence difficult.

In one analysis by Ahluwalia and Doll (1968), death rates from cancer of the cervix in British Columbia were compared with those in the rest of Canada. This particular comparison was chosen because extensive cervical screening had been conducted in British Columbia for longer than in most parts of the world. No significant difference between this and other Canadian provinces was found. Subsequently, a more extensive analysis found that the intensity of cervical screening was associated with a reduction in mortality from cancer of the uterus in Canada during the 1960's for women aged 30 to 64 years (Miller, Lindsay, & Hill, 1976).

At the international level, mortality from cancer of the uterus from 1950 to 1971 was analyzed with a view to estimating the efficacy of screening programs (Hill, 1976). Using World Health Organization data from 58 countries, age-specific death rates for cancer of the cervix and other uterine cancers were calculated for those countries with data available for the period of 1955–1959 to 1965–1969. In all countries but one there was some downward trend in the rate of uterine cancer as a whole. The rates of cervical cancer are too unreliable to be used as they stand, and so the fall in all uterine cancer was arbitrarily chosen as the indicator for the trend in mortality from cancer of the cervix. Countries with a decline of less than 15% in the rate of all uterine cancer were judged unlikely to have had a substantive fall in the rate of cervical cancer. Based on this approach, it was concluded that during the 1960's a significant fall in mortality from cancer of the cervix at ages 35–64 years occurred almost certainly in Canada, New Zealand, and Norway, and probably occurred in Australia, Portugal, Switzerland, and the United States. In order that the relationship of screening to these changes be described, further inferences are required.

During the 1960s cervical screening was introduced on a large scale in countries including the United States and Canada. Although there was a worldwide decline in uterine cancer mortality, this was more marked in some countries, including those with cervical screening. While the effect of screening on this fall in mortality is by no means clear, it seems probable that screening has contributed at least in part to the improvement (Hill, 1976).

Factors other than screening which may have influenced cervical cancer death rates also need to be considered. While active sexual behavior increases the risk of cervical cancer, there is no evidence that this declined during this period; rather, the reverse is more likely. Better genital hygiene has possibly reduced the risk of the transmission of an infective agent. Other possible factors are the more effective treatment of cervical infections and the increased frequency of hysterectomies. Although there have been improvements in treatment during the past 30 years, this is not considered to have been an important contribution to the fall in cervical cancer mortality (Hill, 1976).

General progress towards finding effective treatment for cancer has been surprisingly slow despite the technical sophistication of modern investigative, therapeutic, and surgical methods. Breast cancer and cervical cancer exemplify two diseases for which intervention has some beneficial effect on the course of disease. With cancers such as lung cancer and melanoma, there has been less success, while with Hodgkin's disease and some leukemias, relative cures are now possible. The effectiveness of current therapy is particular to the given cancer even though the molecular causative mechanism appears to be similar for all cancers. Biological knowledge of cancer and the identification of specific causative agents have not yet led to a treatment effective in interrupting disease progression in the majority of cancers.

Cardiovascular Disease

The treatment of cardiovascular disease is generally more encouraging than the present situation for cancer. There have been major advances in the treatment of elevated blood pressure (hypertension) and probably significant developments in the treatment of angina pectoris. Management of heart attacks (myocardial infarction) has been revolutionized, but evidence of the community-level benefits of this are less well substantiated.

Hypertension

Individuals with hypertension are usually free of symptoms. The exception to this is the very small minority with severe elevation of blood pressure who commonly are symptomatic, and therefore present themselves for investigation and treatment. The diagnosis of hypertension can only be done through physical examination by actually measuring the arterial pressure with a blood pressure cuff. This can be initiated by the individual or by a clinician. In the early 1970s in America it was estimated that half of the hypertensives were undetected; that of those identified only half were treated; and that in half of those treated the treatment was inadequate (Pedoe, 1982). This meant that 1 in 8 hypertensives were adequately treated. This situation has changed, with improvement in both case finding and medical therapy.

Community screening for hypertension was originally considered
necessary to identify the large number of undetected cases. When
evaluated, it was found that it would be more effective and efficient
for general practitioners to screen their own patients for hypertension than to conduct special public screening programs. Commonly 70% of the population visit their doctor at least once a
year and 90% within a 5-year period (D'Souza, Swan, & Shannon,
1976). If doctors measured all patients' blood pressure irrespective
of the reason for the consultation, the vast majority of hypertensives would be diagnosed.

After finding an elevated blood pressure, it is necessary to verify
the diagnosis by repeated readings under standard conditions. The
importance of considering the accuracy of diagnosis is discussed
later in this chapter.

The patient with hypertension needs to be linked with a doctor
who will manage treatment on a long-term basis. The effectiveness
of antihypertensive treatment has been well demonstrated through
multiple randomized controlled trials. Medication needs to be taken
throughout life; then the morbid consequences of elevated blood
pressure such as stroke, heart failure, eye disease, kidney disease,
and heart attacks can be reduced significantly.

The largest of the early randomized controlled trials was the
Veterans Administration Cooperative study (1967, 1970). Patients
with diastolic blood pressures ranging from 90 to 129 mmHg were
studied. Initially, treatment for patients with highly elevated diastolic blood pressure, 115 to 129 mmHg, was studied and this
rapidly demonstrated a significant reduction in morbidity. In the
second phase 380 male hypertensive patients with diastolic blood
pressures averaging 90 to 114 mmHg were randomly assigned to
either antihypertensive medication or placebos. Over a 5-year
period, treatment reduced the risk of a serious complication from
55 to 18%. There were half as many deaths from hypertension
or atherosclerosis in the treated group as among the untreated
patients. The effectiveness of treatment was mainly in the reduction
of strokes, congestive heart failure, and renal damage rather than
in preventing heart attacks or sudden death due to coronary heart
disease. In patients with a diastolic pressure above 114 mmHg,
eye complications (hypertensive neuroretinopathy) were also reduced. Treatment also reduced diastolic blood pressure to levels
where the risk of complication was significantly lower. In this
study, the above benefits did not pertain to all degrees of hypertension; a significant improvement was not observed in patients

with a blood pressure below 165/105 mmHg. The next phase of research into antihypertensive therapy was the further investigation of treatment for mild hypertension. The initial results of the Australian Therapeutic Trial (Management Committee, 1979) in mild hypertension found benefits for patients with a diastolic blood pressure above 100 mmHg, but it was with the results of the Hypertension Detection and Follow-up Program (1979) (HDFP) that a new phase in antihypertensive therapy began.

The HDFP (1979) was the first trial to identify the effectiveness of antihypertensive medication for individuals with mild hypertension. This trial included 158,906 people aged 30 to 69 years with diastolic blood pressures ranging upwards from 90 mmHg. The participants were subdivided according to diastolic blood pressure into three strata, 90 to 104 mmHg, 105 to 114 mmHg, and 115 mmHg and above. The patients of each stratum were randomly assigned to receive either Stepped Care (SC) or Referred Care (RC). SC is antihypertensive medication increased stepwise to achieve and maintain the blood pressure at or below set goals. Approved and accepted medications were grouped into five steps so defining the order in which they were to be prescribed if the preceding drug was ineffective in reducing the blood pressure adequately. In contrast to the Veterans Administration Trial (1967, 1970), no one in the study was denied therapy. The patients assigned to RC were referred for treatment to their usual sources of care. The purpose of the trial was to evaluate SC versus RC in terms of reduction in total deaths from all causes. The result was favorable, with all-cause mortality being significantly less in the SC group compared with RC, particularly in patients with a diastolic blood pressure of 90 to 104 mmHg. In this group, the 5-year mortality was 20% lower than in the controls. The authors point out that this finding has enormous potential significance for the community's health. The majority, approximately 70%, of all hypertensives in the population have a blood pressure between 90 and 104 mmHg, and approximately 60% of the excess mortality attributable to high blood pressure overall occurs in individuals with a diastolic pressure in this range. Therefore, the potential number of premature hypertensive deaths which could be avoided through the prescription of and compliance with Stepped Care is very great.

Detection of hypertension and the prescription of efficacious drugs are inadequate unless the patient complies with therapy. Lack of compliance is a significant problem, and much investigation has been conducted to find strategies to improve adherence to prescribed drug regimens. Single strategies such as instruction about the disease or medication, the use of special pill containers, home visits, improving the convenience of care, and monitoring the effect of treatment have all proved ineffective in increasing both antihypertensive drug compliance and the effectiveness of treatment. By contrast, the use of several compliance strategies in combination have proved effective consistently in a number of trials. These compliance packages usually combine various forms of instruction, reinforcement, and monitoring, and have resulted in both improved compliance and improved blood pressure control (Haynes, 1979).

The degree of mastery over hypertension is an achievement for both biomedical science and clinical behavioral science. The combined effect of efficacious pharmacological therapy and successful methods of behavior modification has brought the harmful effects of hypertension closer to eradication than has been accomplished for any other major chronic disease.

Angina Pectoris and Myocardial Infarction

A common and serious symptom of coronary heart disease is pain, angina pectoris, due to insufficient blood flow to the heart muscle. During exercise the demand for oxygenated blood increases, so angina pectoris usually first appears on exertion and is relieved by rest. When one or more of the narrowed coronary arteries supplying the heart muscle become blocked a segment of heart dies or is infarcted (myocardial infarction or heart attack).

In coronary bypass surgery a vein is grafted around the narrowed section of one or more coronary arteries and this allows blood to flow adequately to the previously undernourished heart muscle. This form of surgery is an alternative to drug therapy for angina pectoris. Trials to evaluate the effectiveness of coronary bypass surgery have compared surgery with medical therapy in terms of reducing symptoms and mortality.

In the American Veterans Administration Trial (Read et al., 1978) of surgery for chronic stable angina pectoris, 686 men aged 27 to 67 years were randomly allocated to coronary bypass surgery or medical treatment. Longevity was similar for both groups: 4-year survival was 86% for the surgical group and 83% for the medical group. This similarity was not present for all subgroups, however. Men with left main vessel disease treated surgically had a significantly better survival than those receiving medical therapy.

There was no difference for patients with one and two diseased coronary arteries, although a slight trend in favor of surgery was reported for men with three-vessel disease, but this was not statistically significant. These findings are corroborated by the European Coronary Surgery Study (1980). Among 768 men under 65 years of age with mild to moderate angina, the 5-year survival rate in those randomized to surgery was 93.5%, compared to 84.1% among men assigned to medical treatment. The benefit of surgery was greatest in patients with disease of the left main coronary artery (92.9% vs. 61.7%, 5-year survival) and slightly better among patients with three-vessel disease (94.9% vs. 84.8%). The surgically treated group also was better than the medically treated group in terms of symptomatic improvement, need for medication, and exercise performance.

In the urgent treatment of unstable angina, the American National Cooperative Study Group (Russell et al., 1978) conducted a randomized trial of urgent coronary bypass surgery versus intensive medical management. This study found that relief of pain was similar in the two modes of treatment and that early death and heart attack rates showed no difference.

Positive evidence is now accumulating that coronary bypass surgery is the preferred treatment for a proportion of angina patients, depending upon factors including the nature of symptoms and the underlying coronary disease. Where effective, surgery can offer relief from pain and lower mortality better than medical therapy alone. The widespread use of coronary surgery preceded these research findings rather than being restricted until therapeutic efficacy was established. If this had occurred, coronary operations may have become a more selective procedure than appears to be the case; more than 100,000 coronary bypass operations are performed in the United States each year (Editorial, 1983).

When coronary artery disease advances beyond the stage of angina, further narrowing of coronary vessels results in myocardial infarction. In the first hours following a heart attack the incidence of death is very high, and complications such as arrhythmias and heart failure require rapid attention. Coronary care units (CCU) were developed to manage these problems and to reduce fatality. Although the rationale was sound, CCUs were introduced without prior evaluation (Bloom & Petterson, 1973). One problem demonstrated in the Teeside Coronary Survey (Colling et al., 1976) is that over 70% of deaths occur within 3 hours of onset of a heart attack and the majority of these happen before admission to a CCU.

The first controlled trial of CCUs was started in England in 1966 (Mather et al., 1976). In this study 450 men under 70 years who had suffered a myocardial infarction during the preceding 48 hours were randomly assigned to either home care by their family doctor or hospital care initially in an intensive care unit. They were followed for at least one year. By 28 days 12% had died among those treated at home compared with 14% among the hospital group; and the corresponding death rates at 11 months were 20% and 27%. The authors concluded that home care is a proper form of treatment for many patients with an acute myocardial infarction, particularly those over 60 years of age and those with an uncomplicated attack seen by general practitioners (Hill, Hampton, & Mitchell, 1978). The results of these trials have not been without their skeptical critics, for reasons including the indisputable efficacy of resuscitation methods to avert certain cardiac deaths. The counter argument is that the peak risk of cardiac arrest for the majority of heart attack patients has passed by the usual time of admission to a CCU; and for patients outside hospital, the CCU can do nothing to help until the patient is admitted.

The debate over the impact of CCUs has been heightened by the downward trend in heart disease mortality, as this may be partially attributable to medical care, including CCUs. An attempt to assess the role of hospitals in the decline was made by surveying in-hospital mortality from acute myocardial infarction in all 63 acute care hospitals in the Boston area for 1973–1974 and 1978–1979 (Goldman et al., 1982). No change was found, which is contrary to what would have been expected had hospital care contributed to the 17% decline in American national coronary heart disease mortality which occurred between 1973 and 1978. The impact of CCUs has turned out to be less than was anticipated initially.

The acute care of a myocardial infarction is followed by rehabilitation and long-term management. A number of interventions directed towards factors including smoking, serum cholesterol, and exercise have been evaluated with variable results. In one multifactorial intervention program in Sweden (Vedin et al., 1976) the rate of nonfatal reinfarction was reduced, but only a trend towards improved survival was produced. A Finnish rehabilitation program (Kallio et al., 1979) has been successful in lowering mortality significantly, although the reinfarction rate was higher among patients receiving the multifactorial intervention.

In summary, the treatment of heart disease, and particularly angina and myocardial infarction, is at best a mixture of successes and uncertainty. The prognosis of heart disease patients is very variable and the effectiveness of any form of treatment is influenced by the characteristics of the patients. This is well demonstrated in the case of coronary artery surgery, the effectiveness of which depends upon how the coronary arteries are affected. In general, bypass surgery can alter the prognosis for a proportion of patients. However, the evidence on effectiveness of intensive medical care on heart attack victims has been disappointing, and the course of disease once a myocardial infarction occurs seems to be refractory.

Discussion

The extensive understanding of disease and sophistication of modern treatment methods have contributed to overestimating the strength of medical therapy. With some exceptions, curing disease or even slowing the rate of progression of disorders such as cancer and heart disease are still largely unconquered areas of medicine. The extent of the inadequacy of medical therapy has been illuminated by the use of strict research methods and the use of randomized controlled trials to evaluate the effectiveness of treatment. This experience has led to improvements in research and a greater awareness of factors which heighten the accuracy and usefulness of therapeutic trials.

METHODOLOGY

Evaluations of screening and therapy are open to various pitfalls related to the accuracy of diagnosis. The previous four chapters have concerned populations at risk of disease, while this chapter has dealt with diagnosed diseases. As has been shown, most commonly the outcome of disease depends predominantly upon the disease itself and to a lesser degree upon the effect of medical interventions. In order to identify the effect attributable to intervention, the effect due to the disease itself must be controlled by equalizing its effect in the study group and the control group. This can be done only when the diagnosis is made consistently and accurately in all patients in the study. The methodological issues discussed here relate to various aspects of diagnostic accuracy as this affects evaluation of therapeutic interventions.

Screening

Screening for disease is designed to identify individuals for diagnostic assessment who have not yet consulted a doctor. The hope is that an earlier diagnosis resulting from screening will initiate earlier treatment and an improved prognosis. Irrespective of the benefits of screening, it results in a diagnosis being made sooner than usual. This lead time between the advanced time of diagnosis and the usual time of diagnosis extends the period during which the patient is known to have disease. This longer period can be mistaken to be prolonged survival when it reflects no more than a shift in the time of diagnosis. Trials of screening programs need to correct for lead time ("zero-time shift") in order to assess the true impact of screening on the natural history of diseases (Sackett, 1980).

A second problem in screening concerns the relationship between the length of the preclinical and clinical stages of disease. A disease with a long preclinical phase may also have a long clinical phase, and the converse applies to those with a short preclinical phase. This has been demonstrated for cancers of the lung, breast, and rectum. The longer the preclinical phase, the more likely it is that screening will identify the disease, so screening will favor these diseases rather than those with a more rapid course (Sackett, 1980).

Third, individuals who volunteer for screening may have a better prognosis than those who do not. This was demonstrated in a study, discussed previously, in which women who responded to invitations to attend a mammography clinic had lower mortality from several diseases for which they were neither screened nor treated (Shapiro, 1977).

Clinical Disagreement

Turning to the accuracy of diagnosis the first consideration is the consistency of clinical assessment. A diagnosis is assigned to a patient based on the interpretation of information gathered through history taking, physical examination, tests, and investigations. The long training and extensive experience of doctors would presumably result in considerable clinical consistency between clinicians. Variations have been observed among specialists of the same discipline and in all aspects of clinical assessment. Documented examples are numerous, but some include disagreement between cardiologists over the history of angina pectoris, disagreement in blood pressure reading, and in the interpretation of mammograms and coronary angiograms. Such variability is a combination of inconsistencies between clinicians as well as some degree of individual variability. The importance of clinical disagreement depends upon the clinical circumstances; sometimes clinical disagreement is of major importance and at other times it is inconsequential. In research it is particularly important that observer variation be minimized (Department of Clinical Epidemiology, 1980a).

There are three general sources of clinical disagreement. First, the examiner's performance may vary, in terms of his/her senses, interpretation of his/her perceptions, and categorization of diagnoses. Second, information from the patient may vary either because of actual changes in physical signs or because the patient gives a modified history. Third, the examination itself may give rise to inconsistencies due to disruptive circumstances under which the examination is conducted, or through the incorrect use of diagnostic instruments. A number of strategies to minimize or prevent clinical error have been described (Department of Clinical Epidemiology, 1980b). In research the quality of clinical data should be assessed and specific strategies employed to assure that set standards of consistency are met.

Diagnostic Accuracy

Once the consistency of measurements has been achieved the other major consideration is the accuracy (or validity) of the diagnosis. While consistency is necessary for accuracy, consistency of readings does not guarantee accuracy. For example, two blood pressure readings may be quite consistent but wrong, whereas two correct blood pressure readings must be consistent. There are three dimensions to the accuracy of a test: sensitivity, specificity, and predictive value. Description of these concepts is best done using a two-by-two table such as in Figure 8.1.

The sensitivity of a diagnostic test is the ability to identify correctly individuals with the disease. The margin total, $a + c$, represents the individuals with the disease, and individuals in cell a are those whom the test correctly identifies as positive, so sensitivity = $a/a+c$. The specificity of a diagnostic test is the ability to identify correctly individuals who are free of disease. The margin total, $b+d$, represents the individuals without disease, of whom those in cell d are identified correctly as negative, so

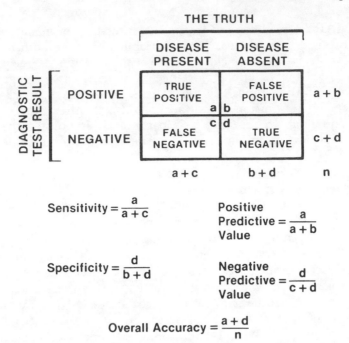

FIGURE 8.1 The accuracy of a diagnostic test.

that specificity $= d/b{+}d$. The sensitivity and specificity of a diagnostic test are constant characteristics and are important for this reason. Of clinical concern, however, is the likelihood that the test result for a given individual is correct. This is the predictive value of the test. Predictive value, different from sensitivity and specificity, varies according to the prevalence of the disease. As the prevalence increases, the likelihood that a positive test result is correct (positive predictive value) increases; and conversely, the likelihood that a negative test result is correct (negative predictive value) decreases.

Even when a randomized trial has been conducted to evaluate a screening program or therapy, there are a number of important methodological pitfalls which need to be considered. The relatively small gains achieved by some therapy requires research methods capable of detecting small increments of change. The numerous sources of diagnostic inaccuracy relevant to trials of therapy and the various design prerequisites for an efficacy trial (Chapter 7) all emphasize the importance of considering the research methods used in a given study in addition to simply reading the results.

SUMMARY

The role of medical therapy in the health of society is less than would be expected, based on the general progress made by biomedical science. The understanding of the biology of disease does not confirm a comparable understanding of medical therapy. In fact, the development of effective medical treatment is a research domain in its own right, which, although facilitated by basic medical science, needs to be evaluated by its own criteria. The decision to implement new therapy should therefore be based on therapeutic trials wherever possible and not only on reasoning extrapolated from basic nonapplied medical research. Even when therapeutic trials have been conducted it is important to scrutinize the exact methods used because trials vary in quality and accuracy. In summary, relatively little is known of the contribution to the health of society made by modern medical and surgical therapy, and in general it seems as though greater potential gains in health are to be achieved through modifying the development of disease than by reversing disease processes after symptoms develop.

Chapter 9

Solutions III: The Role of the Health Care System
Organizational Effectiveness and Efficiency

The treatment of disease used to be a relatively simple procedure, involving little more than an encounter between doctor and patient, but medical care has now grown to involve a vast complex of financial, technical, and professional organizations. Although these organizations have been designed for the effective and efficient delivery of care, these goals are frequently not achieved. Commonly the treatment prescribed lacks efficacy, but this is not the only problem. Other factors such as the organization of services may contribute to diminished therapeutic effectiveness and, unquestionably, the organization of health services is responsible for some of the inefficiencies in health care. In the previous chapter the problems in finding efficacious therapy were described. The contribution of organization to the effectiveness and efficiency of medical care are the topics of this chapter.

The organization of the health care system generally does not influence the choice of medical treatment prescribed (excluding direct government control of medical practice). Organization does, however, affect how services are provided. The first question which will be considered is whether the organization of services can make any difference to the effectiveness of medical treatment. The second section will deal with the evidence that the organization of health services can affect the cost and efficiency of health care.

168

ORGANIZATIONAL EFFECTIVENESS

Introduction

The practical importance of the contribution to health made by organizational structure rests on the extent to which particular organizational characteristics are under our control and can be changed. Decisions such as one to construct a hospital rather than a nursing home, or a rehabilitation program rather than a primary care center, are common decisions in the planning and development of health care. Ideally, the health of the community benefits from such decisions, but this depends upon scientific evidence concerning the effectiveness of these different forms of health care organizations being available to planners. In general terms the organizational components of health care can be grouped into (1) the structural arrangements relating parts to one another; (2) the activities or tasks performed; and (3) the incentives and rewards which motivate the organization to do its job. The latter will be considered mainly in reference to efficiency, whereas the other aspects will be considered in both this section and the next.

Organizational Structure and Health

Type of Health Service

Health care in western society includes a diversity of organizations, many providing care for similar problems. This situation offers the opportunity to compare the relative strengths of different types of organizations, such as group versus solo practice, home care versus hospital care, programmatic organization versus discipline-based organization, and prepaid services versus fee for service. The question is whether these differences matter to the health of the patient.

Group practice reportedly started with the Mayo Clinic in 1884, since which time group practice has developed extensively in both primary and referral practice; many consider it more effective than solo practice. In a comprehensive study of general practice by Peterson et al. (1956) repeated reference is made to the importance of the individual attributes of doctors upon the quality of care. No clear superiority of one form of practice over another was identified; the suggestion that a partnership or group practice had a favorable influence was only sufficient to recommend that this relationship be further investigated. As has been pointed out by Roos (1980) the view that group practice is superior lacks a sound empirical base; study results are inconsistent and data sources problematic. In a study of fee-for-service doctors (Roos 1980), which overcame a number of the methodological inadequacies of previous studies, no differences were observed in therapeutic decisions or clinical outcomes between group and solo practitioners.

As has already been described (Chapter 8), trials have been conducted comparing the efficacy of home and hospital care for patients with acute myocardial infarction (Mather et al., 1976; Hill, Hampton, & Mitchell, 1978). Neither form proved superior, and as Johnson (1980) concludes in a critique of coronary care units, this subject is open for further investigation.

A program of care that is comprehensive and continuous would seem to be more effective than care provided through a variety of uncoordinated services. This assumption was tested with a randomized trial of infant care (Gordis & Markowitz, 1971) in which an integrated hospital-based pediatric program staffed by a pediatrician, a public health nurse, and a social worker was compared with traditional care provided through emergency rooms, well-baby clinics, and outpatient clinics. No differences were observed, following a year of observation, in the completeness of immunization, use of services, morbidity, or mortality.

A further structural variant of health care is prepaid medical service, which differs from private practice in having a contractual responsibility to care for a voluntarily enrolled population. Evaluations of the Health Insurance Plan of greater New York (Shapiro et al., 1960) in the mid-1950s showed prepaid care to be more effective than private practice in terms of permaturity rates and perinatal mortality. The results of later evaluations are less definite. A prospective study of pregnancy outcomes in Oregon (Quick, Greenlick, & Roghmann, 1981) between 1973 and 1974 showed little difference between members of a prepaid service and the general population. Prematurity, neonatal, and infant mortality rates were all similar and only birthweight showed a difference among some patients. The birthweight of newborns whose prenatal care started in the first trimester was 29 grams higher than that of the general population. In sum, from available data, the outcomes from prepaid care are similar or a little better than with conventional care; so the question of the effect of prepaid medical practice on the quality of care remains unresolved (Luft, 1980a).

Specific Aspects of Organization

Within organizations various specific structural components have been studied from the point of view of organizational effectiveness. In a study of 96 American hospitals (Shortell & Logerfo, 1981), a number of organizational features were examined in terms of the quality of care for two conditions: coronary heart disease and appendicectomy for appendicitis. The indicators of quality were mortality among acute myocardial infarct patients, and the rate of normal appendices removed at operation for appendicitis. Interestingly, neither bed size, teaching involvement, nor staff specialty composition were related to quality of care. Some degree of association was observed between quality and organizational variables including the following: doctor participation in hospital decision-making, frequency of committee meetings, the limiting of practice to one hospital, and the proportion of doctors on contract. These findings were not consistent for both conditions. Additionally, the presence of a coronary care unit and a bigger volume of patients were associated with fewer coronary deaths. These results, although statistically significant, should be interpreted cautiously as all these variables combined only explained approximately 15% of the variance in quality of care.

In a review of the organizational determinants of medical care quality, Rhee (1983) has summarized the findings of a wide range of studies. The organizational factors included in the review were the nature of organizational goals, the types of work performed, organizational size, volume of services, extent of division of work (specialization), degree of regulation of work, centralization/decentralization of decision making, integration of work, open evaluation of performance, and medical staff organization. The relationship with the quality of care was inconsistent for all factors except volume of services, specialization, and medical staff organization, for which there were positive associations.

A variety of other aspects of organization have been studied in terms of quality of care. Nurse practitioners and physicians' assistants have been shown to provide care of a quality comparable to that of physicians (Sackett et al., 1974; Sox, 1979). Informational input in the form of continuing medical education was found to increase knowledge but not to alter the quality of clinical practice (Sibley et al., 1982). In a study of innovative clinical behavior, the prescribing of a new drug related to a doctor's associations with other doctors and the clinical behavior of colleagues (Menzel &

Katz, 1955). The quality of care in hospitals, evaluated by process measures of quality, has been observed to depend upon medical school affiliation (Morehead & Donaldson, 1964).

Some General Aspects of Organization

At the most general level of organization McKeown (1979) argues, as has been described previously, that health care has played a relatively minor role in determining the health of society. In promoting health in the population at large McKeown's thesis is that organizational and therapeutic effectiveness have been overshadowed by life style and environmental factors. In a rather novel analysis of mortality in 18 developed countries, Cochrane, St.Leger, and Moore (1978) found a markedly positive association between the prevalence of doctors and mortality. The authors point out that they have no satisfactory explanation for this disquieting observation. Despite large numbers of doctors, medical manpower tends to be maldistributed; doctors congregate in urban and suburban regions leaving the inner city and remote rural areas underserviced. In addition to geographical maldistribution the growth of specialty practice has created an imbalance between the availability of primary care practitioners and consultants (Ontario Economic Council, 1976).

The importance of organizational structure to health varies widely, depending upon the aspect of health and the particular dimension of organizational structure under consideration. In primary care, whether the health care provider is a nurse practitioner or a doctor and whether the practice is group or solo do not appear to be important in terms of quality of service. Conversely, the maldistribution of medical manpower may jeopardize community health by denying access to efficacious treatment. Overall, however, the structural organization of care has not been demonstrated to be a major factor in the effectivenesss of care. In part, this may be due to methodological difficulties in investigating the relationship between structure and outcome. The structure, process, and outcome of health care and the association between these variables have been studied in detail with respect to the evaluation of quality of care. Organizational structure is not thought sensitive as an index of quality due to our inability to observe a close relationship between structure and the effectiveness of care, as this review has shown.

The Process of Care and Health

Similar to the study of organizational structure, assessment of the relationship between clinical performance (process measures) and health outcomes has not yielded results easily understood by the medical profession. Researchers wanting to employ process measures as indicators of quality of care have sought to validate these measures against health outcomes. In an analysis of quality of care for hypertension (Nobrega et al., 1977) no statistical significance was found between 89 process items (including clinical assessment, investigation, treatment, and follow-up) and blood pressure control. Due to the lack of an observed relationship between process and outcome, a controversy has developed over the use of process measures as indicators of quality of care. The considerations are numerous. Although there are accepted standards of management for given diseases, studies of the process of care have not shown that variations in clinical performance adversely affect the patient's health (McAuliffe, 1979).

Availability and Health

Availability is a concept which has been given particular relevance in health care since World War II. The assumption has been commonly made that with access to health services community health would improve and the need for services would diminish. This was Lord Beveridge's philosophy, under which the British National Health Service was introduced. Implicit in this philosophy is the belief that health care is a major determinant of health. The disappointing truth of the small change in health during the first 30 years of the National Health Service is spelled out in the Black Report (Townsend & Davidson, 1982). As described in earlier chapters, community health in Britain did not improve as anticipated and inequalities in health between social classes did not disappear; some inequalities increased. Availability is but one aspect in a number of prerequisites needed before health services can be effective (Sackett, 1980). An efficacious therapy is the first prerequisite. Following this, care must be available and used by the patient. If an efficacious treatment is prescribed, the regimen must be adhered to in order that it be effective.

Patient Compliance with Health Care

To this point, the effectiveness of the health care system has been examined in terms of characteristics of the system itself: organizational structure, performance, and availability. In addition, consideration needs to be given to the patient and the patient's compliance with care. Of treatment prescribed for patients, a large proportion is not followed, and lack of compliance is a significant problem. Keeping appointments may be as low as 50% when initiated by the doctor, except when children are involved, but this rises to 75% when patients request the appointment. With short-term regimens compliance is generally similar in magnitude, ranging from 60 to 80%. The situation in long-term treatment is less favorable, and while variability is considerable, compliance approximates 50%. Adherence to diet is particularly low (Sackett & Snow, 1979). Strategies which have been found effective in improving compliance are summarized in Table 9.1.

"From one perspective, compliance with preventive and therapeutic regimens can be considered a problem in logistics or

TABLE 9.1: Successful compliance-improving strategies

Compliance problem	Strategy
Referrals	Letter to patient
	Referral clerk
	Patient instruction
	(Short referral time)
Appointments	Mailed reminders
	Telephone reminders
	(Efficient clinic scheduling)
Acute medical regimens	Explicit verbal and written instruction
	Parenteral treatment
	Special pill packaging
	Pill calenders
	Extended-role nursing
Chronic medical regimens	Monitored drug levels
	Parenteral medications
	Increased supervision
	Behavior modification
	Physician instruction

From R.B. Haynes. 1979. Strategies to improve compliance with referrals, appointments, and prescribed medical regimens. In R.B. Haynes, D.W. Taylor, and D.L. Sackett (Eds.), *Compliance in health care* (pp. 121–143). Baltimore: Johns Hopkins University Press, p. 142. Reproduced by permission from the Johns Hopkins University Press.

organization" (Gibson, 1979, p. 278). A series of steps to effective clinical management, described initially for the control of hypertension (Task Force on Hypertension, 1978), serves as a guide to understanding the organizational dimension to compliance referred to by Gibson. These steps are, in sequential order, case detection, linkage with care, clinical evaluation, initiation of an efficacious regimen, compliance with treatment, and long-term follow-up and care. Failure of any step jeopardizes the possible benefit of treatment. Implementation of these steps, including multifaceted compliance programs for long-term care (Haynes, 1979), requires an organized system that broadens the focus of health care beyond the traditional role of diagnosis and treatment. Compliance research has emphasized a new type of goal for medical organization, one which is concerned with the patient's behavior and the successful implementation of a broad program for disease management.

Discussion

Many of the studies concerning organizational effectiveness have investigated analytic structural questions such as whether nurse practitioners can provide care of equal quality to that provided by physicians, or whether home care is as good as hospital care for heart attack patients. In general, this type of research has told us that a number of variations in organizational structure are more or less equivalent. By contrast, there has been little medical organization research into questions of how best to meet therapeutic objectives, such as the six steps required for the effective management of hypertension.

Medical organization research most commonly has failed to demonstrate any significant impact on the health of the community. This may be due to several factors. In the first place medical therapy itself does not appear to play a large role in changing the course of disease. Second, it is possible that lack of compliance with efficacious therapy may be responsible for reducing any observable beneficial effects that organizational structure might have on health. Third, medical organization research suffers from at least as many methodological difficulties as clinical research in the areas of strict and appropriate selection of study subjects, achieving reliable measurement of variables, and choosing the type of analysis appropriate to the investigation.

The vast financial outlay on highly expensive medical organizations, for which effectiveness has not been demonstrated, contrasts dramatically with the scientific approach taken in many other domains of medicine. Whether or not organizational structure can directly help the health of the community, one of the most important contributions from organizational research at the present time will be to identify efficient and economic ways to deploy existing resources.

EFFICIENCY OF HEALTH CARE

Introduction

A problem concurrent with effectiveness is the containment of costs of health care within the limits of available resources. Because the resources for the provision of health care are limited, choices need to be made. For each allocation decision an opportunity to spend those same resources in an alternative way is forfeited. For example, government funds allocated to the health sector restrict the funds available for other government departments. Within health the expenditure on professional services defines the amount remaining for other purposes. While there are many similarities between the allocation of health care resources and other sectors of society, the "marketing" and consumption of medical services are quite distinctive. Once someone becomes sick, very little is as important to them as medical care. Usually the patient seeks the available care because he/she needs it, not because he/she can afford it. Decisions on the nature and extent of investigations and therapy, and therefore cost, usually are not made by the patient. The majority of health care costs are determined by the providers of care and the medical technology available to them.

In general terms health care costs depend upon the price of medical goods and services and the quantity consumed. Increases in both prices and the quantity of health care have resulted in large increases in health expenditure. Although part of the price increase is due to inflation, there has also been a true increase in price. Higher medical fees and salaries and more expensive and sophisticated methods of diagnosis, investigation, and treatment have all contributed to the greater price of health care. Increases in the number of doctors, a larger doctor/population ratio, population growth, a greater proportion of elderly people, growth in medical technology, increased patient expectations, and an increased number of services per patient prescribed by the average doctor have all increased the quantity of health care. Many of these changes relate to economic development, so the magnitude of health care expenditure is associated with national wealth. With economic growth the expenditures on health tend to rise.

As national economy differs from country to country so does the amount spent on health. Illustrative of this is the wide international variation in health expenditure per head of population. Health expenditure in 1975, estimated in U.S. dollars, was $226 per person in the United Kingdom, $464 in Australia, $508 in Canada, $607 in the U.S., and $707 per person in Sweden (Maxwell 1981, pp. 29–57). These expenditures have been increasing steadily for the past 25–30 years. The variation in health expenditure correlates broadly with the differences between these countries in gross national product (GNP) per capita. The proportion of the GNP expended on health in 1977 for these countries was, respectively, 5.2%, 7.9%, 7.1%, 9.0%, and 9.8%. These expenses have been dominated by the cost of institutional care, which accounts for 50 to 70% of health expenditure (Maxwell, 1981, pp. 59–96); the expenditure which is accounting for the greatest proportional increases in health costs is that spent on professional services.

The reasons for the rise in costs are multiple and complex. This has led to a search at different levels within the health care system for methods to increase the efficient use of health resources. Of particular concern has been the efficiency of professional services.

Methods

In order to identify efficient ways to employ health resources, several types of economic analysis are employed. Central to these methods is maximization of the benefits from health care and minimization of all costs which are incurred from foregoing the opportunity to make alternative use of resources (opportunity costs). There are two principal outcomes of interest in an economic analysis: the costs of the services and the health benefits.

Conceptually, the simplest form of economic analysis is cost minimization. This involves a simple comparison of costs of two services with identical effectiveness and is designed to identify the more efficient service. When two treatments differ in both their costs and effectiveness a cost-effectiveness analysis is usually indicated. The purpose of such an analysis is to define the cost of the relative effectiveness of one treatment over another (Drummond & Mooney, 1982). In more complex situations when the effects of a treatment are multiple, either cost-benefit or cost-utility analysis can be employed. In cost-benefit analysis the costs and benefits are converted into monetary units so they can be compared directly. An alternative to this is cost-utility analysis, in which benefits are converted into a measure of value or utility, and the cost of a given amount of utility with each treatment is compared.

There are several criteria for assessing the adequacy of an economic analysis (Sackett, 1980). It is important that related costs and benefits are assessed in addition to the direct and obvious effects. For example, costs such as the time patients lose from work in receiving care, and benefits such as the reduced anxiety from minimal delays in obtaining treatment, are important aspects of health care and ideally should be accounted for in a cost analysis. The second major consideration in an economic analysis is a comparison with other ways the same resources could be used. Third, only those services with demonstrated effectiveness should be evaluated. Finally, the measures of cost and benefit need to be credible and the method of analysis appropriate to the question being asked.

Efficiency of Personal Health Services

In the design of some forms of health service economic efficiency is a more prominent concern than in others. For example, in prepaid health programs and in services using nurse practitioners the potential gains in efficiency are of particular interest. The evaluation of some of these services will be described.

Prepaid health plans have been in existence in the United States for over a century, but have grown in prominence with the heightened concern for the cost of health care. In a prepaid plan or health maintenance organization individuals contract with the plan for their medical care for a set period. At the end of the period the contract is renewed if the consumer chooses. Entry into the system is generally made when the individual is well rather than during an illness. It is in the financial interest of the health plan that the individual remains well, and in this way, providers are given an incentive and the opportunity to contain costs by providing quality care.

In terms of the economic evaluation of prepaid health plans the question is whether they are more efficient than conventional fee-for-service medicine. Despite the importance of the question no randomized trials have been conducted to compare the two systems. Added to which, our understanding is limited by the wide diversity of prepaid plans that exist, the variable quality of available data, and the relatively few plans that have been subjected to systematic evaluation with publication of the results (Luft, 1980a). Despite these limitations, available data consistently indicate that the total costs of medical care among the enrollees of health maintenance organizations (HMO) is lower than for conventional care (Luft, 1978). Unfortunately, the evidence does not suggest that the rate of increase in these costs is significantly less than that being observed in medical care in general (Luft, 1980b).

The cost difference between health maintenance organizations and conventional care can arise from either a lower cost per unit of service or from a lower number of services per patient. As HMOs pay the same for medical resources, and as doctors' salaries are similar to those in other sectors, it is probable that differences in utilization explain the lower total costs of HMOs.

Although HMOs probably increase their efficiency to some degree through reduced duplication of services, factors such as organizational size and the use of allied health professionals offer similar benefits to both HMOs and the fee-for-service system and are unaffected by differences in the financing arrangement. The principal gains in cost saving in HMOs appear to relate to differences in the use of services.

Utilization of ambulatory services tends to be higher in HMOs than in conventional care. Hospital usage, however, is lower and this seems to apply to admission rates for all conditions. Observed differences in the use of preventive services do not appear to relate to the type of health care organization as much as it reflects the presence or absence of insurance coverage for preventive visits (Luft, 1980a). Concurrent with the higher ambulatory care utilization in prepaid plans is a greater use of x-rays and laboratory investigations than occurs in conventional care (Hastings et al., 1973). There are therefore both economic advantages and disadvantages associated with prepaid health services; the economic gains tend to be brought about mainly through reduced utilization, principally of hospital beds.

Other strategies have also been successful in reducing hospital utilization. One of these is a variation of prepaid insurance in which private primary physicians are the coordinators and financial managers of all medical care received by their patients. This is a method of cost-containment through risk-sharing (Moore, 1979). The profits and losses are divided between the insurance company and the primary physician. As with an HMO, a commercially and medically viable balance needs to be made between cost-saving and the quality of care. Quality, evaluated by audit, has been found satisfactory and total hospital bed days, admission rates, and length of stay have all been found to be lower than in Blue Cross enrollees. One interpretation of these findings and those of HMO performance is that gains in efficiency are attainable through the use of financial incentives.

The evaluation of efficiency in innovative models of care delivery, which lack cost-containment incentives, provide an interesting contrast to the above. For example, nurse practitioners have been considered as a possible means to increased efficiency in primary care. Their attachment to a practice is a structural change rather than a modification of incentives. Evaluation of the financial impact of nurse practitioners has not shown any clear financial gains, and in fact their presence may bring added costs (Chambers, Bruce-Lockhart, & Black, 1977; Chambers, 1979; Spitzer et al., 1974). In a study by Gordis and Markowitz (1971), mentioned previously, the integration of infant care services into a comprehensive hospital-based program did not affect utilization rates. Any potential cost saving which could have resulted from reduced frequencies of attendance did not occur.

From studies such as these, efficiency in personal health services appears to be related to the incentives given to providers of care rather then to the organizational structure of services. Although doctors receive only a small proportion of the finances spent on health care, they influence the major proportion of health care expenditure. The physicians' decisions concerning the use of services are the major determinants of health care costs.

Interpretation

The increasing costs of health care have led to many proposals and theories concerning cost containment. Many of these lack direct empirical substantiation, while others are supported by scientific evidence. In order to control health expenditure, society has two choices available to it. Either private practice is restructured to establish an effective market system, or responsibility for cost control is taken over by government such that regulation is used in place of incentives. With specific reference to the United States, Walter McClure describes a reciprocal relationship between these two alternatives, so that the fewer the market forces which exist, the stronger the regulatory forces will need to be. He postulates that "if we can have effective market forces in our private system aligned with the objectives of public policy, then the regulation needed to contain cost and to redistribute resources appropriately will be minimal and more likely to work" (McClure, 1978, p. 261).

In countries such as the United States, Canada, and Australia, among others, incentives exist to overutilize health resources. Insurance and government subsidy protect the patient from out-of-pocket expenses, and in most instances the doctor lacks an incentive to consider cost when deciding upon which treatment to offer his/her patient. The availability of numerous and elaborate investigations, medicolegal considerations, and patient expectations all favor overusage. These forces commonly override other medical and economic considerations.

Health insurance without a user fee for each item of medical service removes most of the consumer's incentive to limit cost. Alternatively, if health insurance provided a protection against major medical expenses and left the consumer to pay for the common smaller expenses, then patients would exert a cost control upon their doctors by asking them to avoid unnecessary and expensive management. However, such a plan of strong cost-sharing by consumers, while theoretically sound, probably is not an acceptable proposition (McClure, 1978). The consumer is the prime focus of such a scheme; a more complete approach would include cost-saving incentives for both patients and doctors.

Enthoven's (1978b) proposal of a consumer-choice health plan (CCHP) incorporates cost-saving incentives for consumers and providers of health care. Enthoven (1978a) states that "if the decision makers in a system are not concerned with cost effectiveness, the system will not be cost effective" (p. 652). In the CCHP, the government would change financial incentives by creating a system of competing health plans in which doctors and patients could benefit from using resources wisely. Each health plan would set its own insurance rates and report on its efficiency achievements. A government agency would review such information and make it available to consumers in the community served by the health plan. Individuals would choose their health plan based on the information provided and would than keep the savings from the economy of their choice. In this system the physicians accept responsibility for managing the total health care costs of their enrolled population and thereby retain their professional autonomy.

The alternative to these and other market place methods of cost control is for government to administer or regulate health expenditure. Government regulation can be effective, as demonstrated in Britain. The British government decides on the amount of finances to be allocated to health care. This amount and no more is given to the National Health Service to provide health care to the country. Intrinsic to such an approach is loss of professional autonomy and independence, which is considered abhorrent by many doctors and undesirable by many consumers. In the view of some the initiative will need to be taken by the private sector to make the market approach functional if government regulation is to be avoided (McClure, 1978).

SUMMARY

The organization of health services is a frequent focus in the debate over how best to meet the health needs of society. However, the importance of organizational structure to the effectiveness of health care is not clear. The effectiveness of a variety of services has been evaluated, but no single organizational structure has been identified as superior to another. Similarly, research into the effectiveness of organizational structure in industry has found that there is no single best way to organize (Lawrence & Lorsch, 1967). Research findings concerning the efficiency of health care are somewhat the same in that comparable degrees of efficiency have been achieved by different forms of health service organization. The incentive structure appears to be the single most important organizational feature to cost-containment in a private system. In addition, government administered medicine is capable of controlling costs, and this presents a growing challenge to private medicine to demonstrate that medical costs can be controlled without government regulation. The question of some types of health services being superior for the care of particular diseases has only been investigated in a limited number of instances. As with health care in general, there is evidence that with services for specific diseases there is no single best way to organize.

The organizational structure of health services has not had the thorough evaluation that numerous preventive measures and many medical therapies have received. The beneficial effect of health care results primarily from preventive measures and medical therapy rather than from the variety of organizational designs through which service is provided. The role of an effective organizational structure is to make these services available to the community. The additional role of organization, which is becoming increasingly important, is cost-control. Both the providers of care and consumers can influence the demand for services and the quantity of services consumed. The organizational design can provide cost-saving incentives for both doctors and patients. While an efficient incentive structure has been established in private business a similar arrangement has been slow to develop in private medicine. In countries without nationalized medicine the design and implementation of economic health care organizations may be necessary if government regulation is not going to intervene and convert medical care into another government agency.

Chapter 10

Population Health in
Perspective

The scientific and technical achievements of western society are overwhelmingly impressive by any standards, yet, despite this, much remains outside our control. The often dramatic manner by which medical science is able to relieve pain and suffering has given us hope that biomedical research can provide a solution to all health problems. The evidence presented in the text has shown the problem to be more complex than medical science alone can cure. Some diseases, such as smallpox and hypertension, can be prevented and effectively treated by medical measures. There are many others, such as arthritis, cancer, and strokes, for which health care has brought little change. A number of factors unrelated to medicine influence the development of major chronic diseases and injury, and medical management does not possess effective strategies to cope with much of the existing morbidity and handicap. This book provides a general overview of what we currently know about health. A population perspective serves several important purposes, particularly when striving to achieve a balanced approach to health which is responsive to the needs of a diversified society.

HEALTH AND HEALTH CARE

One of the most important questions to be asked of western society concerns the relationship of health and health care. A health service consisting of a variety of institutions, of which the acute hospital is the most prominent, and staffed with doctors, nurses, and a range of health professionals, has become society's response to the need for health. The world's largest single health care organization, the British National Health Service, was established in 1948 on the premise that as health services are provided to the sick, the society's health will improve and the need for health care will decline. The same philosophy presumably pertains to the many countries spending up to 10% and more of their gross national product on health care. As has been shown most clearly in the case of the first 30 years of the National Health Service in England and Wales, the provision of health care does not alter the need for services. Because of the generally high standard of health enjoyed by so much of western society and the associated sophistication of medical science, these British findings are surprising and unexpected.

Modern health services, based on biological sciences, are principally the product of scientific advances made during the last two centuries. Prior to this era the practice of caring for the sick had been cloaked in myth and dogma, lacking a basis in fact. Understandably, the ravages of tuberculosis, sepsis, and the contagions were surrounded with fear and superstition. These views gradually gave way to a rational view of disease as the discoveries of Pasteur, Semmelweis, Lister, Koch, and the many other contributors to bacteriology developed a scientific explanation for infectious disease. Irrespective of the wide ramifications of disease there was now sound evidence identifying specific microorganisms and precise pathology as the focal cause of morbidity and death. This provided the basis for the reductionist concept that typifies the biomedical view of disease in medical practice today. From the late 19th century new discoveries and their application in practice reinforced the importance of a scientific approach to disease. The medical experience of World War I strengthened this point of view. This was one of the first wars in which deaths from communicable disease were less than those from battle casualties. It has been said that the greatest achievement of the war was in the application and effectiveness of the science of infectious disease in combating disease among the soldiers (Garrison, 1966, p. 790). The use of antitetanus toxoid, typhoid vaccine, antiseptic techniques, x-rays, and improved surgical techniques all contributed to the progress. The period between the world wars saw many more advances. Discoveries such as antibiotics, insulin, antiviral vaccines, and vitamin B-12 expanded the antidisease armamentarium far beyond what could have been anticipated. During World War II the management of casualties brought deformity and death among the

injured to an unprecedented low, and since then surgical achievements have continued to mount. As these developments form
part of the repertoire of modern health services it is understandable
how health care has become equated with health.

Many factors have changed in the course of the 20th century,
making the interpretation of events difficult and often inaccurate.
Whereas the diseases at the turn of the century were largely
infectious in nature, this is no longer so, and now chronic disorders
of heart, lung, brain, and joints predominate. This change has
important implications for treatment. Individuals of all ages were
vulnerable to infectious disease, so for the fortunate who were
cured, many years of relatively healthy life remained. The benefits
of effective treatment were therefore great. With chronic disease,
most patients are middle-aged or older and far fewer years of
potential life remain. Even if a chronic disease is curable the gains
in terms of years of life saved are small. For infectious disease
there is a single microorganism responsible which makes the use
of a specific intervention against the cause a reasonable and effective
means of treatment. To date, the cause of chronic diseases appears
to be multifactorial, and this precludes the use of specific measures
comparable to those used in the treatment of communicable
disorders. Furthermore, our understanding of the cause of many
chronic diseases is very much less than of those caused by bacteria
and parasites. Expectations and values of health and illness are
changing as a result of the altered pattern of diseases and the
chronic nature of disorders such as heart disease, stroke, cancer,
and arthritis. For individuals with an incurable chronic disorder,
their needs become ones of adaptation and adjustment in order
to lead a satisfying life despite the disease. This presents a problem
for a disease-oriented health care system. This is because the
attainment of a level of physical, social, and psychological functioning compatible with a satisfactory quality of life is not the
principal purpose of modern health services. This point will be
expanded upon subsequently. There are therefore a number of
reasons why health care, as presently organized, has been called
into question for not meeting the health problems of today (Illich,
1975; Kennedy, 1980; McKeown, 1979).

The Avoidance of Disease

Evidence has been reviewed (Chapter 7) concerning the reduction
of risks to health including smoking, fatty diet, alcohol con-

sumption, dangerous driving, and immunization against infectious disease. From the data it is evident that the effectiveness of health care in primary prevention varies with the problem that is being prevented. As is made clear by an examination of the occurrence of disease, health care has been highly successful in preventing infectious disease, while chronic diseases have been altered comparatively little. This applies particularly to interventions employed by health professionals such as advice and counseling on smoking, drinking, diet, and road safety. There are, however, some effective preventive interventions that are outside the jurisdiction of the health care system, including price regulation of alcohol and cigarettes and drunk-driving legislation.

Curing Disease

In considering the role of health care in curing disease, it is important to keep in mind that promoting health through treating the sick is the primary function that the modern health care system has chosen and designed for itself. Therefore, it comes as a serious message to society that the general impact of health care on the natural history of disease is small. Admittedly, there are examples of diseases which can be completely cured and others for which the course is greatly improved. Such achievements include the treatment of pneumonia, meningitis, hypertension, many surgical conditions, insulin-dependent diabetes, schizophrenia, pernicious anemia, Hodgkin's disease, and others. There remain, however, the major causes of death—cancer, heart disease, and stroke—for which the improvements from medical treatment are modest or negligible.

Reducing Morbidity

The third means by which health care can influence health is through reducing morbidity and suffering. The effectiveness of rehabilitative, supportive, and palliative therapy has not been reviewed in the text but needs to be referred to at this point. Orthopedics, plastic surgery, and other surgical specialties have made important contributions to the reduction in pain, deformity, and disfigurement and to the improvement of physical mobility. Rehabilitation medicine has trained large numbers of handicapped individuals to adapt to their physical and mental limitations. Many specialties within the health professions are involved in the long-term care of patients whose primary disease or disability cannot be cured but who need help coping and adjusting to life. Family physicians and psychiatrists spend larger portions of their time helping people with problems which interfere with daily activities. In fact, most of us have experienced a time when the services of an understanding health professional could have made us feel better. The quality of life, whether physical, social, or psychological, is a major function of health care; however, scientific evaluation of the impact of health care on quality of life is sparse, and we can only speculate as to the effectiveness of this aspect of clinical practice.

In these three areas of health care there is a wide variation in the extent to which modern medicine benefits health. The relationship is inconsistent, and in terms of chronic disease there is no strong indication that health care, in its present form, is going to play a major part in eradicating the major chronic diseases. There is, however, extensive scientific evidence identifying a number of life style and environmental factors that play an important part in causing disease (Chapters 5 and 6). The task for society is to clearly identify the source of today's health problems, to develop methods to remove the hazards, and to maintain and develop the effective components of the health care system. These tasks provide a rational basis for health policy.

SCIENCE AND HEALTH POLICY

The formulation of health policy is a political process and as such is subject to a variety of influences. Financial and economic expediency and considerations of influence and control are commonly major determinants of policy. Scientific evidence, if it exists, is often overshadowed by these other considerations. As more scientific data on health are made available, biased decisions will be more difficult to make. By employing scientific methods the population perspective on health aims to produce a global definition of health problems and solutions, and thus provide an unbiased and objective basis for health policy.

A national health policy in the form of explicit objectives and priorities has more to do with an ideal state than with actual practice. By comparison, other types of government policy like trade, defense, or international aid are more explicit and more easily recognizable than policies to promote health. Because chronic disease and accidents are caused by life style and environmental factors, an effective health policy would need to involve the jurisdiction of many government departments, including at least education, agriculture, urban development, the environment, communication, social services, and transportation. The common form of health policy is one dominated by the administration of health services and health insurance. In order that steps be made towards improving a nation's health, policies need to be formulated concerning such major problems as poor nutrition, accidents, cancer, cardiovascular health, and social and emotional isolation.

A rational policy requires a sound information system. In the case of health, as the previous chapters have illustrated, the quality, diversity, and availability of health information presents many challenges and inadequacies. Special attention is needed to establish a scientific data base for health policy.

Identification and Description of Health Problems

The first component of a scientific information system should be a method for the identification and description of health problems. Aspects of this can be easily overlooked. The general improvement in society's health has fostered a belief that good health is shared equally by everyone. This is not so, particularly for groups such as the elderly, the poor, the socially isolated, some ethnic groups, the disabled, those with certain diseases, and the geographically isolated. National health should be defined both at the level of the whole population and within specific subgroups in order to identify inequalities. A mechanism for analyzing population health data in this way would allow such information to be routinely available.

In order that all types of health problems are recognized and brought to the attention of decision makers, the data collected on community health should include morbidity as well as mortality. Death rates and the causes of death are recorded routinely. However, the consequences of disease and data on psychological and social handicap are poorly documented despite their importance. Once society has reached a high degree of development, statistics on life expectancy and some mortality rates, such as infant mortality, show little change and are of little use for new policies. New forms of data are required to adequately define new problems. Descriptive epidemiological methods have been used to define the frequency distribution of disease in the population; these methods should be applied to study morbidity resulting from chronic disease and injury. Knowledge of the epidemiology of disability and handicap will provide an essential step in the search for ways to reduce illness and improve the quality of life.

Research into the Origins of Illness, Handicap, and Disease

Very commonly the morbidity seen in clinical practice cannot be fully explained on the basis of a recognizable disease. Symptoms such as concern, worry, pain, and incapacity are very often poorly understood and inadequately treated. This is frustrating to both the patient and the person treating the patient. The cause of disease has been the focus of research for centuries but there is a need for a new form of etiological research. We need to understand why some individuals suffer from incapacitating symptoms while others do not. Why can one heart attack victim cope with life while a patient with a similar disease is incapacitated with fear and apprehension? Can these people be helped? Is their problem genetic, or are there factors such as exercise, education, training, or social contact which can help them? Although the treatment of disabling symptoms is of major concern to patients, symptomatology in its own right is an insignificant subject in Western medicine. In order to find factors, other than specific diseases, which predispose to illness, both handicap and illness need to be the focus of analytic research.

Research into the Effectiveness and Efficiency of Interventions

Growth in knowledge of pathological processes and mechanisms of disease has repeatedly led to new forms of treatment being implemented for which effectiveness has been assumed and not tested. Despite their biological logic many major forms of treatment have been found to be either ineffective or no more beneficial than an alternative treatment. Some examples include bed rest for myocardial infarctions, gastric freezing for bleeding in the upper gastrointestinal tract, radical mastectomy for cancer of the breast, and coronary care units for heart attack patients. In times of sophisticated technology and vast medical research activities the potential for generating new forms of treatment is considerable. In the interest of avoiding harm to patients, in investing energy into beneficial measures, and in containing costs, it is necessary that new forms of treatment be thoroughly evaluated before going into general use. Both therapeutic effectiveness and economic efficiency should be assessed.

The process of defining problems, investigating causes, and testing solutions is a continuous process. Once measures have been implemented to resolve a problem, the step of assessing the frequency and distribution of the problems in the community should be repeated. Refinements and modifications of all stages of this cycle will need to occur as problems, evidence, and technology change.

The science of medicine and health care has largely been exclusive to health professionals and scientists. If health policy is to compete with other national policies for priority then the health issues at stake and the relevant evidence need to become known to the public at large. Evidence concerning the health of the population should be part of general education and not limited to the tertiary training of medical specialists.

THE PATIENT AND HEALTH CARE

In the course of the technical evolution of medicine the profession's view of the patient has changed. The patient's own perception and experience has become progressively less the focus of attention as the doctor's technical interaction with the patient's disease has grown in sophistication and intensity. Is the patient himself of interest to health professionals, or is the patient simply the bearer of an interesting disease? This question can be asked of all aspects of the health field, of the educational institutions, of the organization of health services, and of the way services are provided.

Medical education has been the domain of medical specialists for most of this century, so it is not surprising that the medical school curriculum is primarily a reflection of specialized medical practice. Significant changes have occurred, however, which have introduced both behavioral science and general practice into medical training. Behavioral sciences are commonly taught by social scientists and not physicians. One can wonder whether physicians feel unprepared to teach medical students about patient behavior and doctor–patient communication, or whether the delegation of behavioral science to social scientists served to safeguard the role of academic physicians (Harper, 1971). Nevertheless, so long as teaching behavioral science fails to involve clinical role models little practical changes can be hoped for. The doctors who teach students tend not to be selected because of their knowledge and interest in the comprehensive care of individuals; rather, they are expert in the management of particular diseases. A balance among clinical teachers would assure that students are exposed to generalists and specialists and that they are taught to treat both patient and disease.

Underlying this discussion is the question of whether society wants doctors to be responsible for more than the treatment of disease. If so, then there are many health problems affecting patients for which doctors are ill prepared to manage. If doctors are to treat patients as well as diseases then one can ask why patients are not used in medical schools to teach students about the problems of patients. Patients are routinely used to demonstrate the signs and symptoms that are of interest to doctors, but how often are they asked to demonstrate problems of concern to patients? Similarly, if the environment and the patient's functioning within his/her environment are important components of illness, how can students be taught to care for patients without teaching taking place in the patient's home environment? Hospitals are excellent places to learn about the health care system and disease but they teach us little about patients as ordinary people.

An important reason for the slow and modest change towards broadening medical education has been the lack of knowledge and research into health problems beyond the disease itself. Consequently, few professionals have been considered sufficiently competent in the clinical application of behavioral sciences to develop this area of medical education. General practice has been largely a nonacademic discipline, but with research and the development of academic training general practice may be in a position to do for patient management what specialized medicine has done for the treatment of disease.

The organization of the health care system may be able to compensate for some of the shortcomings of specialization. Departmentalization of services has fragmented patient care, separating one specialty from another and generalist from specialist. General practitioners work in the community near to patients yet often removed from specialized services, and specialists congregate in large medical facilities which house the elaborate technology of medicine. Little interaction occurs between the two. This fragmented arrangement denies hospital-based specialty practice the advantages of the generalist's perspective and starves general practice of the benefits of specialist input. The patient needs to learn what services he/she can expect form the different parts of the system, knowing that his/her care will rarely be coordinated and packaged for his/her convenience. If the health care system were more service oriented and designed to help the patient, it would be organized differently. The role of the nurse would be developed to give her/him greater responsibility and flexibility in responding to the needs of patients and to facilitating the coordination of services. The allied health professions such as occupational therapy, physiotherapy, and speech therapy would also be used to increase the comprehensiveness of care. General practitioners and nurses would be expected to coordinate patient care, and reciprocal consultation between specialists, general practitioners, and nurses would occur routinely and on a regular basis. General practitioners would visit hospitals and specialists would visit communities. Generalists and specialists would collaborate in and share academic activities.

The ultimate test of the responsiveness of the health care system is the quality of the encounter between doctor and patient. The comprehensiveness of the care provided rests on the doctor's ability to respond to the patient's concerns while at the same time providing appropriate medical management of disease. This is not an easy task as doctors have acquired the role of controlling the doctor-patient relationship and of arbitrating over the presence of legitimate illness. This control has risen from the doctor's extensive medical knowledge of disease and the many criteria he or she applies in order to make a diagnosis. However, in addition to disease the patient has problems of a subjective and idiosyncratic nature which, to the patient, oftentimes outweigh the importance of any accompanying disease. In order that these problems be treated, the doctor must accept the patient's concerns in their own right and act upon them as bona fide problems, without judgment. The doctor's adaptation to the patient's perception of problems is an essential element in the provision of comprehensive care (Harper, 1974), although this is not a skill in which the doctor is formally trained. Frequently, the patient is frustrated by the doctor's preoccupation with medical concerns and apparent disinterest in how the patient feels.

The needs of patients will always be difficult to meet. Our individuality gives us the creativity to solve most of our own problems, but our idiosyncrasy is also responsible for a limitless variety of needs and problems that are a continuing challenge to the providers of human services.

A POPULATION PERSPECTIVE ON HEALTH

In the course of this volume, I have aimed to illustrate the value of what I have called a population perspective on health. This has involved a speedy journey through a number of aspects of the medical literature. Now that this is done, you may well ask how can we make use of this approach. The evidence and methods of this population perspective that have been described form the basis for my proposal, which follows. The action needed is not exclusive to any sector or group, whether professional or lay. We should all take responsibility to develop a particular view of health and integrate it into our lives. I suspect, however, that thinking with a population perspective may develop more slowly among professionals in the health field than in the rest of society. The community would gain considerably in terms of health if it were to encourage those responsible for the health of society to adopt an approach to health which integrates the individual and community perspectives.

Past experience with infectious disease has taught us to think of health in terms of specific causative agents. In recent decades specialization in medicine has isolated one aspect of medical practice from another. This has evolved to the degree that psychiatrists treat the mind, podiatrists the feet, and in between are more than 50 specialties attending their own segmented domain of human health. This isolationism serves the interests of the providers of care, and is reflected in the piecemeal nature of educational curriculums, financing systems, and the organization of health services. In contrast to this fragmentation, the health problems of patients are characterized by interdependence with one another, and by interdependence with life style and environment. The interrelatedness of the numerous aspects of health have been a recurring theme throughout the data presented and affect the occurrence of disease, the use of health services, and the impact of illness on everyday life. Body and mind do not function separately. Health is influenced by the environment, and the environment is affected by the health status of the people living in it. Our behavior affects our health, and our physical, emotional, and social functions affect how we live and think.

The fragmented way in which we have conceptualized our health system has not been a fully conscious feature in the architectural design of health organizations. This has developed more by default and oversight than by a deliberate plan to isolate the structure and function of the various parts of the health system. In order that this separateness be overcome, we need to understand the interdependencies which are important to health and to develop strategies to facilitate exchange and reciprocity. This is the first of five essential components to a unified population perspective.

Questions of how to incorporate health strategies into fields outside health have arisen largely by crisis and confrontation, and not by forethought and design. Occupational health and safety legislation in industry, drunk-driving legislation, and antismoking regulation exemplify this reactive rather than active approach. Strategies are needed to integrate health protective measures into public policies. National food and agriculture policies present a difficult challenge to the development of a national nutrition policy that is needed to promote health in terms of fighting coronary heart disease, cancer, diabetes, and obesity. A problem of similar magnitude exists for commercial policies affecting the control, advertising, and sale of alcohol and cigarettes. A health policy to control the health effects of alcohol and cigarettes continues to be overshadowed by commercial interests. The health component of public policies concerning housing, urban development, transportation, education, communications, and the media illustrates the need for a national health policy that by necessity should be incorporated into nearly all public policies.

Within the health field the problems of overlapping priorities and interests are also very complex. The curricula for health professions reflect the fragmentation which characterizes health care. Very few educational programs integrate disciplines, such as occurs in the problem-based method of teaching. The shared responsibilities of a consulting physician and a consultant are aspects of medical organization which can be described as laissez-faire at best. Symptomatic of organizational fragmentation are the formal barriers separating specialty and general practice, as occurs in Britain and Australia.

Integration and coordination are the domain of systems analysts. These functions have been studied extensively in industry for purposes of improving business profits and productivity. Reciprocity and coordination in the health field for purposes of improving health have not been given comparable attention. The interdependency of health with other aspects of society, and the correspondence between areas within the health field, constitute the linkage points at which the diverse components of population health are brought together. This integration and coordination is needed to convert a plan for health into action. This all starts from investigation of the linkages that are necessary and from an understanding of the function which the coordination of health activities will bring.

Throughout my description of population health I have endeavored to demonstrate the importance of accurate documentation. The ease with which false conclusions about health can be drawn is so great that the use of strict criteria for the evaluation of evidence must be an intrinsic component of a population perspective. Epidemiology and biostatistics provide this numerical approach which is essential for objectivity in health decisions.

The third element in a population perspective concerns how humans see themselves and value their own way of life. Emphasis has been placed on the subjective experience of health and illness and the need to complement an objective assessment of health with the feelings and views of the patient. Health and sickness cannot be fully understood without taking an anthropological perspective. This involves consideration of the beliefs, customs, and values of the patient as well as the family and group to which the patient belongs. While some contact with unfamiliar ethnic and religious customs is not an uncommon experience for many health professionals, adaptation to health beliefs, customs, and values is not generally a formal part of our health care system. The scientific disease orientation of medicine precludes this. Attitudes toward such questions as abortion, occupational safety, pollution, and smoking are becoming well publicized due to action taken by public lobby groups. There is yet to develop a formally recognized dimension of medical practice that involves the assessment of the patient's view of his or her illness. An anthropological perspective in this context does not concern the study of rare and unusual tribes; it is concerned with understanding the individuals and groups who are treated everyday. This perspective on health includes the ethical issues of health care as well as the customs governing how policies are made and implemented.

One of the dilemmas of health in western society, which I described at some length, is the unequal distribution of illness across different groups in the population. Many subgroups of society have quite distinctive health experiences, associated with which are differing health needs. Added to this are inequalities in the distribution and availability of services. Health varies with education, income, occupation, race, age, sex, geographical location, social contacts, the presence of disease, and disability, among other factors. Some of these groups may well be less able to make use of facilities than others; for example, new immigrants and the functionally illiterate may be unable to read hazard warning signs and protective directions. Access to health care may also vary due to bias and discrimination. In order that inequities be reduced or avoided, the principles of distributive justice need to form one component of the population perspective. Bias and injustice are ubiquitous in human history and it would be naive to imagine that they can be eliminated. Inequalities in health, however, are a major problem in western society today. If something is to be done to change this situation these inequalities must be identified explicitly and positive efforts made for their amelioration. For this to occur the principle of justice is a necessary element in our approach to health.

A major reason for this book has been the growing discordance between the specific focus of medical services and the diverse and general nature of the health problems affecting society. Biomedical science takes the reductionist view that disease stems from a single cause. Within this framework, the thrust of medical endeavor is tightly focused on particular disease processes. While physical disease itself can be defined in precise pathological terms and often localized accurately within particular systems of the body, this perspective does not include the many functional, psychological, social, and environmental dimensions of illness. The association of occupation, life style, personality, social relationships, income, age, race, and sex, for example, does not come within the reductive view of disease. The point of proposing a population perspective to health is to broaden the definition to include the many factors relating to illness. This wider view of illness helps explain why modern efforts to combat chronic disease and accidents have been unimpressive in terms of their effectiveness. This wider view, however, is not simply the addition of a lens with a wide angle; it is the philosophical converse of the reductionist view.

The fifth and final component to a population perspective is a holistic view of health. An intrinsic feature of this holism is identification of the general class of which individual cases are specific examples. Individual patients are identified as one of a group, or members of a particular population. The patient's presenting complaint is likewise one of a population of symptoms. The patient may complain explicitly of pain but may be reluctant to disclose symptoms of fear, guilt, or impending doom. Also within this broad comprehensive perspective can be included the four preceding dimensions of a population perspective: the systems approach, the numerical view, the anthropological dimension, and distributive justice. None of these characteristics are any more than a tool or instrument, and their effectiveness depends upon how they are used.

The health care systems of western society, designed to treat current disease, have had limited success in improving the community's health. In order to develop an effective approach to illness a strategy is needed that is sufficiently comprehensive to encompass the multiple causes and consequences of chronic disorders. The breadth of these issues dictates that the responsibility for health cannot rest solely with health professionals but must be shared by society in general. This book has set out a framework for analyzing health issues based on consideration of the frequency and distribution of disease and sickness, the factors predisposing to illness, and the effectiveness of interventions. This approach incorporates a community-wide definition of the problem with consideration of individual patients. A population perspective is not a discrete discipline or specialty; rather, it is a general approach to understanding health issues. The breadth and lack of bias that this offers can help us work innovatively and efficiently towards attaining an equitably healthy and fulfilled society.

References

Ableson J, Paddon P, and Strohmenger C. 1983. *Perspective on Health.* Catalogue 82–540E Occasional. Ottawa, Canada: Ministry of Supply and Service.

Ahluwalia HS, and Doll R. 1968. Mortality from cancer of the cervix in British Columbia and other parts of Canada. *British Journal of Preventive and Social Medicine* 22:161–164.

Allgaier E. 1964. *Driver Education Reduces Accidents and Violations* (No.3782). Washington, D.C.: American Automobile Association.

American Heart Association Committee Report. 1980. Risk factors and coronary disease, a statement for physicians. *Circulation* 62(2):449A–455A.

Anderson D. 1967. Road safety on the snowy mountains: Scheme and its application to the community. *Medical Journal of Australia* 1:58–59.

Antonovsky A. 1967. Social class, life expectancy and overall mortality. *Milbank Memorial Fund Quarterly* 45(2):31–73.

Armstrong BK. 1977. The role of diet in human carcinogenesis with special reference to endometrial cancer. In *Origins of Human Cancer,* HH Hiatt, JD Watson, JA Winsten, eds., pp. 557–565. New York: Cold Spring Harbour Laboratory.

Armstrong ML. 1976. Regression of atherosclerosis. In *Atherosclerosis Reviews 1,* R Paoletti and AM Gotto, Jr., eds., pp. 137–182. New York: Raven Press.

Armstrong ML, Warner ED. 1971. Morphology and distribution of diet-induced atherosclerosis in rhesus monkeys. *Archives of Pathology* 92:395–401.

Auerbach O, Hammond EC, and Garfinkel L. 1979. Changes in bronchial epithelium in relation to cigarette smoking, 1955–1960 versus 1970–1977. *New England Journal of Medicine* 300(8):381–386.

Backett EM, and Johnston AM. 1959. Social patterns of road accidents in children, some characteristics of vulnerable families. *British Medical Journal* 1.409–413.

Barron BA, and Richart RM. 1970. A statistical model of the natural history of cervical carcinoma. II. Estimates of the transition time from dysplasia to carcinoma in situ. *Journal of the National Cancer Institute* 45:1025–1030.

Basu TK, Donaldson D, Jenner M, Williams DC, and Sakula A. 1976. Plasma vitamin A in patients with bronchial carcinoma. *British Journal of Cancer* 33:119–121.

199

Baum SG, and Litman N. 1979. Mumps virus. In *Principles and Practice of Infectious Disease*, GL Mandell, RG Douglas, and JE Bennett, eds., pp.1176-1185. New York: John Wiley & Sons.

Beeson PB. 1980. Changes in medical therapy during the past half century. *Medicine* 59(2):79-99.

Benfari RC. 1981. The multiple risk factor intervention trial (MRFIT). III. The model for intervention. *Preventive Medicine* 10:426-442.

Belloc NB, and Breslow L. 1972. Relationship of physical health status and health practices. *Preventive Medicine* 1:409-421.

Bennett L, Hamilton R, Neutel CI, Pearson RJC, and Talbot B. 1977. Survey of persons with multiple sclerosis in Ottawa, 1974-75. *Canadian Journal of Public Health* 68:141-147.

Berkman LF, and Syme SL. 1979. Social networks, host resistance, and mortality, a nine-year follow-up study of Alameda County residents. *American Journal of Epidemiology* 109(2):186-204.

Bjelke E. 1975. Dietary vitamin A and human lung cancer. *International Journal of Cancer* 15:561-565.

Blackburn H, and Gillum RF. 1980. Heart Disease. In *Maxcy-Rosenau Public Health and Preventive Medicine*, Eleventh Edition, JM Last, ed., pp.1168-1201. New York: Appleton-Century-Crofts.

Blazer DG. 1982. Social support and mortality in an elderly community population. *American Journal of Epidemiology* 115:684-694.

Bloom BS, and Peterson OL. 1973. End results, cost and productivity of coronary-care units. *New England Journal of Medicine* 288(2):72-77.

Boyd JH, and Weissman MM. 1982. Epidemiology. In *Handbook of Affective Disorders*, ES Paykel, ed., pp.109-125. New York: Guilford Press.

Brody EM. 1977. Environmental factors in dependency. In *Care of the Elderly, Meeting the Challenge of Dependency*, AN Exton-Smith and G Evans, eds., pp. 81-95. New York: Grune and Stratton.

Buell P, and Dunn JE. 1965. Cancer mortality among Japanese Issei and Nisei of California. *Cancer* 18:656-664.

Burke DC. 1973. Spinal cord injuries and seat belts. *Medical Journal of Australia* 2:801-806.

Burkitt DP. 1969. Related disease-related cause? *Lancet* 2:1229-1231.

Cairns J. 1978. *Cancer, Science and Society*. San Francisco: WH Freeman and Company.

Carvalho AC, Colman RW, and Lees RS. 1974. Platelet function in hyperlipoproteinemia. *New England Journal of Medicine* 290:434-438.

Cassel J. 1977. The relation of the urban environment to health, toward a conceptual frame and a research strategy. In *The Effect of the Man-Made Environment on Health and Behavior*, LE Hinkle and WC Loring, eds., pp.129-142. DHEW Pub. No.(CBC) 77-8318. Washington, D.C.: U.S. Government Printing Office.

Chambers LW. 1979. Financial impact of family practice nurses on medical practice in Canada. *Inquiry* 16:339-349.

Chambers LW, Bruce-Lockhart P, and Black DP. 1977. A controlled trial of the impact of the family practice nurse on volume, quality, and cost of rural health services. *Medical Care* 15:971–981.

Christopher PJ, MacDonald PA, Murphy AM, and Buckley PR. 1983. Measles in the 1980's. *Medical Journal of Australia* 2(10):488–491.

Coburn D, Torrance GM, and Kaufert JM. 1983. Medical dominance in Canada in historical perspective, the rise and fall of medicine. *International Journal of Health Services* 13(3):407–432.

Cochrane AL. 1972. *Effectiveness and Efficiency*. Abingdon Berks: Nuffield Provincial Hospitals Trust.

Cochrane AL, St. Leger AS, and Moore F. 1978. Health services 'input' and mortality 'output' in developed countries. *Journal of Epidemiology and Community Health* 32:200–205.

Colez A, and Blanchet M. 1981. Disability trends in the United States population 1966–76, analysis of reported cases. *American Journal of Public Health* 71(5):464–471.

Colling A, Dellipiani AW, Donaldson RJ, and McCormack, P. 1976. Teesside coronary survey, an epidemiological study of acute attacks of myocardial infarction. *British Medical Journal* 2:1169–1172.

Comfort A. 1979. *The Biology of Senescence*, Third Ed. New York: Elsevier.

Committee of Principal Investigators. 1978. A co-operative trial in the primary prevention of ischaemic heart disease using clofibrate. *British Heart Journal* 10:1069–1118.

Conger JJ, Miller WC, Rainey RV. 1966. Effects of driver education, the role of motivation, intelligence, social class, and exposure. *Traffic Safety Research Review* 10:67–71.

Dalos NP, Rabins PV, Brooks BR, and O'Donnell P. 1983. Disease activity and emotional state in multiple sclerosis. *Annals of Neurology* 13(5):573–577.

Davis DL, and Magee BH. 1979. Cancer and industrial chemical production. *Science* 206:1356–1358.

Dawber TR. 1980. *The Framingham Study, The Epidemiology of Atherosclerotic Disease*. Cambridge: Harvard University Press.

Dayton S, Pearce ML, Goldman H, et al. 1968. Controlled trial of a diet high in unsaturated fat for prevention of atherosclerotic complications. *Lancet* 2:1060–1062.

Department of Clinical Epidemiology and Biostatistics, McMaster University. 1980a. Clinical disagreement, 1. How often it occurs and why. *Canadian Medical Association Journal* 123:449–504.

Department of Clinical Epidemiology and Biostatistics, McMaster University. 1980b. Clinical disagreement, 2. How to avoid it and how to learn from one's mistakes. *Canadian Medical Association Journal* 123:613–617.

Department of Clinical Epidemiology and Biostatistics, McMaster University. 1981a. How to read clinical journals, 3. To learn the clinical course and prognosis of disease. *Canadian Medical Association Journal* 124:869–872.

Department of Clinical Epidemiology and Biostatistics, McMaster University. 1981b. How to read clinical journals, 4. To determine etiology or causation. *Canadian Medical Association Journal* 124:985–990.

Department of Health, Education and Welfare. 1964. *Smoking and Health, Report of the Advisory Committee to the Surgeon General of The Public Health Service.* Public Health Service Pub. No. 1103. Washington, D.C.: U.S. Government Printing Office.

Department of Health, Education and Welfare. 1979. *Smoking and Health, A Report to The Surgeon General.* DHEW Pub. No. (PHS) 79–50066. Public Health Service. Washington, D.C.: U.S. Government Printing Office.

Doll R. 1978. Atmospheric pollution and lung cancer. *Environmental Health Perspectives* 22:23–31.

Doll R. 1980. The epidemiology of cancer. *Cancer* 45(10):2475–2485.

Doll R. 1983. Prospects for prevention. *British Medical Journal* 286(6363):445–453.

Doll R, and Hill AB. 1950. Smoking and carcinoma of the lung, preliminary report. *British Medical Journal* 2:739–748.

Doll R, and Peto R. 1976. Mortality in relation to smoking, 20 years' observations in male British doctors. *British Medical Journal* 2:1525–1536.

Doll R, and Peto R. 1981. *The Causes of Cancer.* Oxford: Oxford Medical Publications.

Doll R, Vessey MP, Beasley RW, et al. 1972. Mortality of gasworkers, final report of a prospective study. *British Journal of Industrial Medicine* 29:394–406.

Donovan JW. 1977. Randomized controlled trial of anti-smoking advice in pregnancy. *British Journal of Preventive and Social Medicine* 31:6–12.

Donovan JW, Burgess PL, Hossack CM, and Yudkin GD. 1975. Routine advice against smoking in pregnancy. *Journal of The Royal College of General Practitioners* 25:264–268.

Drummond MF, and Mooney GH. 1982. Essentials of health economics, part V. Assessing the costs and benefits of treatment alternatives. *British Medical Journal* 285:1561–1563.

D'Souza MF, Swan AV, and Shannon DJ. 1976. A long-term controlled trial of screening for hypertension in general practice. *Lancet* 1(7971):1228–1231.

Eaton WW, and Kessler LG. 1981. Rates of symptoms of depression in a national sample. *American Journal of Epidemiology* 114(4):528–538.

Editorial. 1983. Coronary bypass surgery—here to stay. *Lancet* 2(8343):197–198.

Edsall G. 1959. Specific prophylaxis of tetanus. *Journal of The American Medical Association* 171(4):417–427.

Edwards G, Orford J, Egert S, et al. 1977. Alcoholism. A controlled trial of "treatment" and "advice". *Journal of Studies on Alcohol* 38(5):1004–1031.

Eisinger RA. 1972. Psychosocial predictors of smoking behaviour change. *Social Science and Medicine* 6:137–144.

Elian M, and Dean G. 1983. Need for and use of social and health services by multiple sclerosis patients living at home in England. *Lancet* 1(8333):1091–1093.

Enthoven AC. 1978a. Consumer-choice health plan, (first of two parts) Inflation and inequity in health care today: alternatives for cost control and an analysis of proposals for national health insurance. *New England Journal of Medicine* 298:650–658.

Enthoven AC. 1978b. Consumer-choice health plan, (second of two parts) A national-health-insurance proposal based on regulated competition in the private sector. *New England Journal of Medicine* 298:709–720.

European Coronary Surgery Study Group. 1980. Prospective randomized study of coronary artery bypass surgery in stable angina pectoris, second interim report. *Lancet* 2(8193):491–495.

Falk HL, Kotin P, and Mehler A. 1964. Polycyclic hydrocarbons as carcinogens for man. *Archives of Environmental Health* 8:721–730.

Fanning DM. 1967. Families in flats. *British Medical Journal* 4:382–386.

Farquhar JW, Maccoby N, Wood PD, et al. 1977. Community education for cardiovascular health. *Lancet* 1(8023):1192–1195.

Ferris BG. 1978. Health effects of exposure to low levels of regulated air pollutants, a critical review. *Journal of the Air Pollution Control Association* 28(5):482–497.

Ferris BG, Chen H, Puleo S, and Murphy RLH. 1976. Chronic non-specific respiratory disease in Berlin, New Hampshire, 1967 to 1973. A further follow-up study. *American Review of Respiratory Disease* 113(4):475–485.

Fletcher CM, Peto R, Tinker C, et al. 1976. *The Natural History of Chronic Bronchitis and Emphysema.* Oxford: Oxford University Press.

Ford AB. 1976. *Urban Health in America.* New York: Oxford University Press.

Frank GC, Berenson GS, and Webber LS. 1978. Dietary studies and the relationship of diet to cardiovascular disease risk factor variables in 10-year-old children, the Bogalusa heart study. *American Journal of Clinical Nutrition* 31:328–340.

Freidson E. 1970. *Profession of Medicine.* New York: Dodd Mead and Co.

Friedman GD, Ury HK, Klatsky AL, Siegelaub AB. 1974. A psychological questionnaire predictive of myocardial infarction: results from the Kaiser-Permanente epidemiologic study of myocardial infarction. *Psychosomatic Medicine* 36:327–343.

Fries JF, and Crapo LM. 1981. *Vitality and Aging, Implications of the Rectangular Curve.* San Francisco: Freeman and Company.

Garfinkel L. 1980. Cancer mortality in non-smokers, prospective study by the American Cancer Society. *Journal of the National Cancer Institute* 65:1169–1173.

Garrison FH. 1966. *An Introduction to the History of Medicine,* Fourth Edition. Philadelphia: Saunders.

Gerrity RG. 1981. Transition of blood-borne monocytes into foam cells in fatty lesions. *American Journal of Pathology* 103:181–190.

Gibson ES. 1979. Compliance and the organization of health services. In *Compliance in Health Care,* RB Haynes, DW Taylor, and DL Sackett, eds., pp. 278–285. Baltimore: Johns Hopkins University Press.

Gibson ES, Martin RH, and Lockington JN. 1977. Lung cancer mortality in a steel foundary. *Journal of Occupational Medicine* 19:807–812.

Glasgow Royal Infirmary, Medical Division. 1973. Early mobilization after uncomplicated myocardial infarction prospective study of 538 patients. *Lancet* 2(7825):346–349.

Glueck CJ, and Conner WE. 1978. Diet-coronary heart disease relationships reconnoitered. *American Journal of Clinical Nutrition* 31:727–737.

Glueck CJ, Mattson F, and Bierman EL. 1978. Sounding boards, diet and coronary heart disease, another view. *New England Journal of Medicine* 298(26):1471–1474.

Goldman L, Cook F, Hashimoto B, Stone P, Muller J, and Loscalzo A. 1982. Evidence that hospital care for acute myocardial infarction has not contributed to the decline in coronary mortality between 1973–1974 and 1978–1979. *Circulation* 65(5):936–942.

Goldstein JL, Kita T, and Brown MS. 1983. Defective lipoprotein receptors and atherosclerosis, lessons from an animal counterpart of familial hypercholesterolemia. *New England Journal of Medicine* 309(5):288–296.

Gordis L, and Markowitz M. 1971. Evaluation of the effectiveness of comprehensive and continuous pediatric care. *Pediatrics* 48(5):766–776.

Gordon T. 1970. *The Framingham Diet Study, Diet and the Regulation of Serum Cholesterol, The Framingham Study, an Epidemiological Investigation of Cardiovascular Diseases*. Section 24. Department of Health, Education and Welfare. Washington, D.C.: U.S. Government Printing Office.

Gordon T, Castelli W, Hjortland MC, Kannel WB, and Dawber TR. 1977. High density lipoprotein as a protective factor against coronary heart disease. *American Journal of Medicine* 62:707–714.

Gordon T, Garcia-Palmieri MR, Kagan A, Kannel WB, and Schiffman J. 1974. Differences in coronary heart disease mortality in Framingham, Honolulu and Puerto Rico. *Journal of Chronic Diseases* 27:329–344.

Griffin WV, Mauritzen JH, and Kasmar JV. 1969. The psychological aspects of the architectural environment, a review. *American Journal of Psychiatry* 125(8):1057–1062.

Hammond EC, Selikoff IJ, and Seidman H. 1979. Asbestos exposure, cigarette smoking and death rates. *Annals of the New York Academy of Sciences* 330:473–490.

Harper AC. 1971. The social scientist in medical education, the specialist's safeguard. *Social Science and Medicine* 5:663–665.

Harper AC. 1974. Towards a job description for comprehensive health care, a framework for education and management. *Social Science and Medicine* 7:985–995.

Harper AC, Harper DA, Chambers LW, Cino PM, and Singer J. 1986. An epidemiological description of physical, social and psychological problems in multiple sclerosis. *Journal of Chronic Diseases* 39(4):305–310.

Harpur JE, Conner WT, Hamilton M, et al. 1971. Controlled trial of early mobilization and discharge from hospital in uncomplicated myocardial infarction. *Lancet* 2:1331–1334.

Hastings JE, Mott FD, Barclay A, et al. 1973. Prepaid group practice in Sault Ste. Marie, Ontario. I. Analysis of utilization records. *Medical Care* 11(2):91–103.

Hayes, MJ, Morris GK, and Hampton JR. 1974. Comparison of mobilization after two and nine days in uncomplicated myocardial infarction. *British Medical Journal* 3:10–13.

Haynes RB, 1979. Strategies to improve compliance with referrals, appointments, and prescribed medical regimens. In *Compliance in Health Care*, RB Haynes, DW Taylor, and DL Sackett, eds., pp. 121–143. Baltimore: Johns Hopkins University Press.

Health and Welfare Canada. 1976. *Alcohol Problems in Canada, A Summary of Current Knowledge*. Ottawa: Non-Medical Use of Drugs Directorate.

Health and Welfare Canada. 1982. *Medical Services Annual Review, 1980*. Ottawa: Ministry of Supply and Services, Canada.

Health and Welfare Canada. 1983. *Medical Services Annual Review, 1981*. Ottawa: Ministry of Supply and Services, Canada.

Henderson DA. 1976. The eradication of smallpox. *Scientific American* 235(4):25–33.

Henderson M, and Wood R. 1973. Editorial. Compulsory wearing of seat belts in New South Wales, Australia, an evaluation of its effects on vehicle occupant deaths in the first year. *Medical Journal of Australia* 2:797–801.

Henry SA. 1947. Occupational cutaneous cancer attributable to certain chemicals in industry. *British Medical Bulletin* 4:389–401.

Hill AB. 1977. *A Short Textbook of Medical Statistics*. London: Hodder and Stoughton.

Hill GB. 1976. Cancer of the uterus, mortality trends since 1950. *WHO Chronicle* 30:188–193.

Hill JD, Hampton JR, and Mitchell JR. 1978. A randomized trial of home-versus-hospital management for patients with suspected myocardial infarction. *Lancet* 1(8069):837–841.

Hirayama T. 1979. Diet and cancer. *Nutrition and Cancer* 1(3):67–81.

Hirayama T. 1981. Non-smoking wives of heavy smokers have a higher risk of lung cancer, a study from Japan. *British Medical Journal* 282:183–185.

Hjermann I, Velve Byre K, Holme I, and Leren P. 1981. Effect of diet and smoking intervention on the incidence of coronary heart disease. Report from the Oslo Study Group of a randomized trial in healthy men. *Lancet* 2(8259):1303–1310.

Hollingsworth TH. 1965. A demographic study of the British ducal families. In *Population in History*, DV Glass and DE Eversley, eds., pp. 354–378. London: Edward Arnold.

Hutchinson GB. 1960. Evaluation of preventive services. *Journal of Chronic Diseases* 2:497–508.

Hutter AM, Sidel VW, Shine KI, and DeSanctis RW. 1973. Early hospital discharge after myocardial infarction. *New England Journal of Medicine* 288:1141–1144.

Hypertension Detection and Follow-up Program Cooperative Group. 1979. Five-year findings of the hypertension detection and follow-up program; I, Reduction in mortality of persons with high blood pressure, including mild hypertension. *Journal of the American Medical Association* 242:2562-2571.

Illich I. 1975. *Medical Nemesis, The Exploration of Health*. London: Calder and Boyars.

Jenkins CD. 1976a. Recent evidence supporting psychologic and social risk factors for coronary disease (first of two parts). *New England Journal of Medicine* 294(18):987-994.

Jenkins CD. 1976b. Recent evidence supporting psychologic and social risk factors for coronary disease (second of two parts). *New England Journal of Medicine* 294(19):1033-1038.

Johnson AL. 1979. Fashion and fact in cardiology. Annual Canadian Cardiovascular Society Lecture, 18 October 1979, Montreal.

Johnson AL. 1980. The coronary care unit. *Annals of The Royal College of Physicians and Surgeons of Canada* 13(3):207-210.

Joint Standing Committee on Road Safety. 1982. *Stay Safe I, Alcohol, Other Drugs and Road Safety*. First Report. Parliament of New South Wales. Sydney: D West Government Printer.

Jose DG. 1979. Dietary deficiency of protein amino-acids and total calories on development and growth of cancer. *Nutrition and Cancer* 1(3):58-63.

Kallio V, Hamalainen H, Hakkila J, and Luurila OJ. 1979. Reduction in sudden deaths by a multifactorial intervention programme after acute myocardial infarction. *Lancet* 2(8152):1091-1094.

Kark JD, Smith AH, Switzer BR, and Hames CC. 1981. Serum vitamin A (Retinol) and cancer incidence in Evans County, Georgia. *Journal of the National Cancer Institute* 66:7-16.

Kasl SV. 1977. The effects of the residential environment on health and behavior, a review. In *The Effect of the Man-Made Environment on Health and Behaviour*, LE Hinkle and WC Loring, eds., pp. 65-127. DHEW Pub. No. (CDC) 77-8318. Washington, D.C.: U.S. Government Printing Office.

Kelsey JL. 1979. A review of the epidemiology of human breast cancer. *Epidemiologic Reviews* 1:74-109.

Kennedy I. 1980. *The Reith Lectures: Unmasking Medicine*. The Listener. London: BBC Publications.

Keys A. 1980. *Seven Countries, A Multivariate Analysis of Death and Coronary Heart Disease*. Cambridge: Harvard University Press.

Kuller LH. 1980. Editorial: Prevention of cardiovascular disease and risk factor intervention trials. *Circulation* 61:26-28.

Kuller L, Meilahn E, Townsend M, and Weinberg G. 1982. Control of cigarette smoking from a medical perspective. *Annual Review of Public Health* 3:153-178.

Kurtzke JF. 1970. Neurological impairment in multiple sclerosis and the disability status scale. *Acta Neurologica Scandinavica* 46:493-512.

Lacour J, Lacour F, Spira A, et al. 1984. Adjuvant treatment with polyadenylic-polyuridylic acid in operable breast cancer, updated results of a randomized trial. *British Medical Journal* 288:589-592.

Lalonde M. 1974. *A New Perspective on the Health of Canadians*. Ottawa: Health and Welfare, Canada.

Last JM. 1980. Housing and health. In *Preventive Medicine and Public Health*, Eleventh Edition, JM Last, ed., pp. 864-871. New York: Appleton-Century-Crofts.

Lawrence PR, Lorsch JW. 1967. *Organization and Environment, Managing Differentiation and Integration*. Boston: Harvard University.

Leacy FH, Ed. 1983. *Historical Statistics of Canada*, Second Edition. Ottawa: Statistics, Canada.

Levin ML, Goldstein H, and Gerhardt PR. 1950. Cancer and tobacco smoking, a preliminary report. *Journal of the American Medical Association* 143:336-338.

Levine SA, and Lown B. 1951. The "chair" treatment of acute coronary thrombosis. *Transactions of the Association of American Physicians* 64:316-317.

Lew EA, and Garfinkel L. 1979. Variations in mortality by weight among 750,000 men and women. *Journal of Chronic Diseases* 32:563-576.

Lilienfeld AM, Levin ML, Kessler II. 1972. *Cancer in the United States*. Cambridge: Harvard University Press.

Lipid Research Clinics. 1984. Coronary primary prevention trial, results I and II. *Journal of the American Medical Association* 251(3):351-374.

Lipkin M Jr, Lybrand WA. 1982. *Population-Based Medicine*. New York: Praeger Publishers.

Luft HS. 1978. How do health maintenance organizations achieve their "savings"? Rhetoric and evidence. *New England Journal of Medicine* 298:1336-1343.

Luft HS. 1980a. Assessing the evidence on HMO performance. *Milbank Memorial Fund Quarterly, Health and Society* 58(4):501-536.

Luft HS. 1980b. Trends in medical care costs, do HMOs lower the rate of growth? *Medical Care* 18(1):1-16.

MacMahon B. 1981. Cancer. In *Preventive and Community Medicine*, Second Edition, DW Clark and B MacMahon, eds., pp. 451-468. Boston: Little Brown and Company.

MacMahon B, Cole P, and Brown J. 1973. Etiology of human breast cancer, a review. *Journal of the National Cancer Institute* 50:21-42.

Mahley RW, Weisgraber KH, Bersot TP, and Innerarity TL. 1978. Effects of cholesterol feeding on human and animal high density lipoproteins. In *High Density Lipoproteins and Atherosclerosis*, AM Gotto, NE Miller, and MF Oliver, eds., pp. 149-176. Amsterdam: Elsevier.

Mallory GK, White PD, and Salcedo-Salgar J. 1939. The speed of healing of myocardial infarction, a study of the pathological anatomy in seventy-two cases. *American Heart Journal* 18:647-671.

Management Committee. 1979. Initial results of the Australian therapeutic trial in mild hypertension. *Clinical Science* 57(Supplement 5):449s-452s.

Mann C. 1926. *Diets for Boys During the School Age*. Medical Research Council, London, His Majesty's Stationery Office, Special Report No. 105.

Mann G. 1977. Diet-heart, end of an era. *New England Journal of Medicine* 297:644-650.

Marmot MG, Rose G, Shipley MJ, and Thomas BJ. 1981. Alcohol and mortality, a U-shaped curve. *Lancet* 1(8220 Part 1):580-583.

Marmot MG, Syme SL. 1976. Acculturation and coronary heart disease in Japanese-Americans. *American Journal of Epidemiology* 104(3):225-247.

Marmot MG, Syme SL, Kagan A, Kato H, Cohen JB, and Belsky J. 1975. Epidemiologic studies of coronary heart disease and stroke in Japanese men living in Japan, Hawaii and California. Prevalence of coronary and hypertensive heart disease and associated risk factors. *American Journal of Epidemiology* 102(6):514-525.

Marshall CL. 1980. Prevention and health education. In *Maxcy–Rosenau Preventive Medicine and Public Health*, Eleventh Edition, JM Last, ed., pp. 1113-1132. New York: Appleton-Century-Crofts.

Maslow AH, and Mintz NL. 1956. Effects of esthetic surroundings, I. Initial effects of three esthetic conditions upon perceiving "energy" and "well-being" in faces. *Journal of Psychology* 41:247-254.

Mather HG, Morgan DC, Pearson NG, et al. 1976. Myocardial infarction, a comparison between home and hospital care for patients. *British Medical Journal* 1:925-929.

Maxwell RJ. 1981. *Health and Wealth, An International Study of Health-Care Spending*. Lexington, Massachusetts: Lexington Books.

Mazess RB, and Forman SH. 1979. Longevity and age exaggeration in Vilcabamba, Equador. *Journal of Gerontology* 34(1):94-98.

McAuliffe WE. 1979. Measuring the quality of medical care: process versus outcome. *Milbank Memorial Fund Quarterly, Health and Society* 57(1):118-152.

McClure W. 1978. Choices for medical care. *Minnesota Medicine* 61(4):261-271.

McDermott FT, Hughes ES. 1982. Compulsory Blood Alcohol Testing of Road Crash Casualties in Victoria, the second three years (1978-1980). *Medical Journal of Australia* 1(7):294-296.

McDermott W. 1978. Medicine, the public good and one's own. *Perspective on Biology and Medicine* 21(2):167-187.

McGill HC Jr. 1968. *Geographic Pathology of Atherosclerosis*. Baltimore: Williams and Wilkins.

McGill HC, McMahon CA, Wene JD. 1981. Unresolved problems in the diet-heart issue. *Arteriosclerosis* 1:164-176.

McKeown T. 1976. *The Modern Rise of Population*. London: Edward Arnold.

McKeown T. 1979. *The Role of Medicine*. Princeton: Princeton University Press.

McKeown T, and Lowe CR. 1966. *An Introduction to Social Medicine*. Oxford: Blackwell Scientific Publications.

McNeer JF, Wagner GS, Ginsburg PB, et al. 1978. Hospital discharge one week after acute myocardial infarction. *New England Journal of Medicine* 298:229-232.

Medical Research Council. 1959. Vaccination against whooping-cough. British Medical Journal 1:994–1000.

Medical Research Council. 1977. Clinical trial of live measles vaccine given alone and live vaccine preceded by killed vaccine. Lancet 2(8038):571–575.

Menzel H, Katz E. 1955. Social relations and innovation in the medical profession, the epidemiology of a new drug. Public Opinion Quarterly 19:337–352.

Mettlin C, Graham S, and Swanson M. 1979. Vitamin A and lung cancer. Journal of The National Cancer Institute 62:1435–1438.

Miettinen M, Turpeinen O, Karvonen MJ, et al. 1972. Effect of cholesterol-lowering diet on mortality from coronary heart-disease and other causes. A twelve-year clinical trial in men and women. Lancet 2:835–838.

Miller AB, Lindsay J, Hill GB. 1976. Mortality from cancer of the uterus in Canada and its relationship to screening for cancer of the cervix. International Journal of Cancer 17:602–612.

Miller AB, and Bulbrook RD. 1982. Screening, detection, and diagnosis of breast cancer. Lancet 1(8281):1109–1111.

Miller LW, Older JJ, Drake J, and Zimmerman S. 1972. Diphtheria immunization, effect upon carriers and the control of outbreaks. American Journal of Diseases of Children 123:197–199.

Ministry of Health. 1982. Survey of Non-Institutionized Physically Handicapped Persons in Ontario. Toronto: Government of Ontario.

Ministry of Transportation and Communications. 1981. Ontario Motor Vehicle Accident Facts, 1981. Toronto: Safety Co-ordination and Development Office.

Mintz NL. 1956. Effects of esthetic surroundings, 2. Prolonged and repeated experience in a "beautiful" and an "ugly" room. Journal of Psychology 41:459–466.

Moncada S, and Vane JR. 1979. Archidonic acid metabolites and the interactions between platelets and blood-vessel walls. New England Journal of Medicine 300(20):1142–1147.

Moore S. 1979. Cost containment through risk-sharing by primary-care physicians. New England Journal of Medicine 300(24):1359–1362.

Morehead MA, Donaldson RS. 1964. A Study of the Quality of Hospital Care Secured by a Sample of Teamster Family Members in New York City. New York: Columbia University, School of Public Health and Administrative Medicine.

Morris JN, Chave SP, Adam C, Sirey C, Epstein L, and Sheehan DJ. 1973. Vigorous exercise in leisure-time and the incidence of coronary heart disease. Lancet 1:333–339.

Morris JN, Heady JA, Raffle PA, Roberts CG, and Parks JW. 1953. Coronary heart disease and physical activity of work. Lancet 2:1053–1057.

Moser J. 1979. Prevention of alcohol-related problems, developing a broad-spectrum programme. British Journal of Addiction 74:133–140.

Multiple Risk Factor Intervention Trial Research Group. 1982. Risk factor changes and mortality results. Journal of the American Medical Association 248(12):1465–1477.

Nagi SZ. 1976. An epidemiology of disability among adults in the United States. *Milbank Memorial Fund Quarterly* 54(4):439–467.

National Center for Health Statistics. 1981. Characteristics of nursing home residents, health status, and care received. *Vital and Health Statistics*, Series 13, No. 51. DHHS Pub. No. (PHS)81–1712. Public Health Service. Washington, D.C.: U.S. Government Printing Office.

National Center for Health Statistics. 1982. Current estimates from The National Health Interview Survey, United States, 1981. *Vital and Health Statistics*, Series 10, No.141. DHHS Pub. No.(PHS)82–1569. Public Health Service. Washington, D.C.: U.S. Government Printing Office.

National Center for Health Statistics. 1983a. *Health, United States, 1983*. DHHS Pub. No.(PHS)84–1232. Public Health Service. Washington, D.C.: U.S. Government Printing Office.

National Center for Health Statistics. 1983b. Disability days, United States, 1980. *Vital and Health Statistics*, Series 10, No. 143. DHHS Pub. No. (PHS)83–1571. Public Health Service. Washington, D.C.: U.S. Government Printing Office.

National Center for Health Statistics. 1983c. Patterns of ambulatory care in general and family practice, The National Ambulatory Medical Care Survey, United States, January 1980–December 1981. *Vital and Health Statistics*, Series 13, No. 73. DHHS Pub. No. (PHS)83–1734. Public Health Service. Washington, D.C.: U.S. Government Printing Office.

National Center for Health Statistics. 1984a. *Vital Statistics of The United States, 1979*, Vol. 2, Mortality, Part A. DHHS Pub. No. (PHS)84–1101. Public Health Service. Washington, D.C.: U.S. Government Printing Office.

National Center for Health Statistics. 1984b. Utilization of short-stay hospitals, United States, 1982 annual summary. *Vital and Health Statistics*, Series 13, No. 78. DHHS Pub. No. (PHS)84–1739. Public Health Service. Washington, D.C.: U.S. Government Printing Office.

National Center for Health Statistics. 1984c. Trends in nursing and related care, homes and hospitals, United States, selected years 1969–80. *Vital and Health Statistics*, Series 14, No. 30. DHHS Pub. No. (PHS)84–1825. Public Health Service. Washington, D.C.: U.S. Government Printing Office.

National Center for Health Statistics. 1984d. *Health, United States, 1984*. DHHS Pub. No. (PHS)85–1232. Public Health Service. Washington, D.C.: U.S. Government Printing Office.

National Center for Health Statistics. 1984e. Health indicators for Hispanic, black and white Americans. *Vital and Health Statistics*, Series 10, No. 148. DHHS Pub. No. (PHS)84–1576. Public Health Service. Washington, D.C.: U.S. Government Printing Office.

Nichols AB, Ravenscroft C, Lamphiear DE, and Ostrander LD. 1976. Independence of serum lipids and dietary habits, the Tecumseh study. *Journal of the American Medical Association* 236:1948–1953.

Nobrega FT, Morrow GW, Smoldt RK, and Offord KP. 1977. Quality assessment in hypertension analysis of process and outcome methods. *New England Journal of Medicine* 296(3):145–148.

Nordoy A. 1981. Lipids and thrombogenesis. *Annals of Clinical Research* 13:50–61.

Nordoy A, Refsum N, Thelle D, and Jaeger S. 1979. Platelet function and serum high density lipoproteins. *Thrombos Haemostas* 42(4):1181–1186.

Nordoy A, Strom E, Gjesdal K. 1974. The effect of alimentary hyperlipaemia and primary hypertriglyceridaemia on platelets in man. *Scandinavian Journal of Haematology* 12:329–340.

Office of Population Censuses and Surveys. 1974. Morbidity statistics from general practice, second national study 1970–71. *Studies on Medical and Population Subjects*, No. 26. London: Her Majesty's Stationary Office.

Oliver MF. 1980. Primary prevention of coronary heart disease, an appraisal of clinical trials of reducing raised plasma cholesterol. *Progress in Cardiology* 9:1–24.

Oliver MF. 1981. Diet and coronary heart disease. *British Medical Bulletin* 37(1):49–58.

Ontario Economic Council. 1976. *Health, Issues and Alternatives*. Toronto.

Paffenbarger RS, Wing AL, and Hyde RT. 1978. Physical activity as an index of heart attack risk in college alumni. *American Journal of Epidemiology* 108(3):161–175.

Palmer WG, and Scott WD. 1981. Lung cancer in ferrous foundary workers, a review. *American Industrial Hygiene Association Journal* 42:329–340.

Pedoe HT. 1982. Hypertension. In *Epidemiology of Diseases*, DL Miller and RD Farmer, eds., pp. 122–135. Oxford. Blackwell Scientific Publications.

Peterson OL, Andrews LP, Spain RS, and Greenberg BG. 1956. An analytical study of North Carolina practice 1953–1954. *Journal of Medical Education* 31:1–146.

Peto R, Doll R, Buckley JD, and Sporn MB. 1981. Can dietary beta-carotene materially reduce human cancer rates? *Nature* 290:201–208.

Phillips RL. 1975. Role of life-style and dietary habits in risk of cancer among Seventh-Day Adventists. *Cancer Research* 35:3513–3522.

Pitot HC. 1979. Biological and enzymatic events in chemical carcinogenesis. *Annual Review of Medicine* 30:32–35.

Plant MA, Pirie F, and Kreitman N. 1979. Evaluation of the Scottish health education unit's 1976 campaign on alcoholism. *Social Psychiatry* 14:11–24.

Pooling Project Research Group. 1978. Relationship of blood pressure, serum cholesterol, smoking habit, relative weight and ECG abnormalities to incidence of coronary events; final report of the Pooling Project. *Journal of Chronic Diseases* 31:201–306.

Popham RE, Schmidt W, and de Lint L. 1975. The prevention of alcoholism, epidemiological studies of the effects of government control measures. *British Journal of Addiction* 70:125–144.

Pott P. 1775. *Chirurgical Observations Relative to the Cataract, Polypus of the Nose, the Cancer of the Scrotum, the Different Kinds of Ruptures and the Mortification of the Toes and Feet*. London: L Hawes, W Clarke, and R Collins.

Quick JD, Greenlick MR, and Roghmann KJ. 1981. Prenatal care and pregnancy outcome in an HMO and general population. A multivariate cohort analysis. *American Journal of Public Health* 71(4):381–390.

Read RC, Murphy ML, Hultgren HN, and Takaro T. 1978. Survival of men treated for chronic stable angina pectoris, a cooperative randomized study. *Journal of Thoracic and Cardiovascular Surgery* 75(1):1–12.

Reynolds I, Rizzo C, and Gallagher H. 1981. The prevalence of psychosocial problems, a study of 37,678 Sydney adults. *Australian Family Physician* 10(9):732–741.

Rhee S. 1983. Organizational determinants of medical care quality, a review of the literature. In *Organization and Change in Health Care Quality Assurance*, RD Luke, JC Krueger, and RE Modrow, eds., pp. 127–146. Rockville: Aspen Publications.

Rinzler SH. 1968. Primary prevention of coronary heart disease by diet. *Bulletin of the New York Academy of Medicine* 44:936–949.

Robertson LS, Kelly AB, O'Neill B, Wixom CW, Eisworth RS, and Haddon W. 1974. A controlled study of the effect of television messages on safety belt use. *American Journal of Public Health* 64(11):1071–1080.

Robertson LS, and Zador PL. 1978. Driver education and fatal crash involvement of teenaged drivers. *American Journal of Public Health* 68(10):959–965.

Rogot E, and Murray JL. 1980. Smoking and causes of death among U.S. veterans, 16 years of observation. *Public Health Reports* 95(3):213–222.

Rokin ID. 1981. Etiology and epidemiology of cervical cancer. In *Current Topics in Pathology*, Volume 70: *Cervical Cancer*, G Dallenbach-Hellweg, ed., pp. 81–110. Berlin: Springer-Verlag.

Roos NP. 1980. Impact of the organization of practice on quality of care and physician productivity. *Medical Care* 28(4):347–359.

Rose G, and Hamilton PJ. 1978. A randomized controlled trial of the effect on middle aged men of advice to stop smoking. *Journal of Epidemiology and Community Health* 32:275–281.

Rosenman RH, Brand RJ, Jenkins CD, Friedman M, Straus R, and Wurm M. 1975. Coronary heart disease in the Western Collaborative Group Study, final follow-up experience of 8.5 years. *Journal of the American Medical Association* 233:872–877.

Ross HL. 1981b. *Deterring the Drinking Driver, Legal Policy and Social Control.* Lexington, MA: Lexington Books.

Ross R. 1981a. George Lyman Duff Memorial Lecture. Atherosclerosis, a problem of the biology of arterial wall cells and their interactions with blood components. *Arteriosclerosis* 1(5):293–311.

Rowe G, and Norris MJ. 1985. *Mortality Projections of Registered Indians, 1982 to 1996.* Ottawa: Ministry of Indian Affairs and Northern Development, Canada.

Royal College of General Practitioners' Oral Contraceptive Study, 1977. Mortality among oral contraceptive users. *Lancet* 2(8041):727–731.

Royal College of Physicians. 1971. *Smoking and Health Now.* London.

Russell MA. 1974. Realistic goals for smoking and health. A case for safer smoking. *Lancet* 1:254-258.

Russell RO, Resnekov L, Wolk M, et al. 1978. Unstable angina pectoris, national cooperative study group to compare surgical and medical therapy. *American Journal of Cardiology* 42:839-848.

Sackett, DL. 1979. Bias in analytic research. *Journal of Chronic Diseases* 32:51-63.

Sackett DL. 1980. Evaluation of health services. In *Maxcy-Rosenau Public Health and Preventive Medicine*, Eleventh Edition, JM Last, ed., pp. 1800-1823. New York: Appleton-Century-Crofts.

Sackett DL, and Snow JC. 1979. The magnitude of compliance and non-compliance. In *Compliance in Health Care*, RB Haynes, DW Taylor, and DL Sackett, eds., pp. 11-22. Baltimore: Johns Hopkins University Press.

Sackett DL, Spitzer WO, Gent M, et al. 1974. The Burlington randomized trial of the nurse practitioner, health outcomes of patients. *Annals of Internal Medicine* 80(2):137-142.

Sackett DL, and Whelan G. 1980. Cancer risk in ulcerative colitis, scientific requirements for the study of prognosis. *Gastroenterology* 78:1632-1635.

Salk J, and Salk D. 1978. Vaccination against poliomyelitis. In *New Trends and Developments in Vaccines*, A Voller and H Friedman, eds., pp. 117-153. Baltimore, MD: University Park Press.

Shannon HS. 1982. *Categorization of Statements on Asbestos Related Diseases*. Hamilton: McMaster University, Department of Clinical Epidemiology and Biostatistics.

Shaoul J. 1975. *The Use of Accidents and Traffic Offenses as Criteria for Evaluating Courses in Driver Education*. Salford, England: University of Salford.

Shapiro S. 1977. Evidence on screening for breast cancer from a randomized trial. *Cancer* 39 (Supplement):2772-2782.

Shapiro, S, Jacobziner H, Densen PM, and Weiner L. 1960. Further observations on prematurity and perinatal mortality in a general population and in the population of a prepaid group practice medical care plan. *American Journal of Public Health* 50:1304-1317.

Shattil SJ, Bennett JS, Coleman RW, and Cooper RA. 1977. Abnormalities of cholesterol-phospho-lipid composition in platelets and low-density lipoproteins in human hyperbeta-lipoproteineima. *Journal of Laboratory Clinical Medicine* 89:341-353.

Shepherd DI. 1979. Clinical features of multiple sclerosis in north-east Scotland. *Acta Neurologica Scandinavica* 60:218-230.

Shortell SM, and Logerfo JP. 1981. Hospital medical staff organization and quality of care, results for myocardial infarction and appendectomy. *Medical Care* 19:1041-1055.

Sibley JC, Sackett DL, Neufeld V, Gerrard B, Rudnick KV, and Fraser W. 1982. A randomized trial of continuing medical education. *New England Journal of Medicine* 306(9):511-515.

Smith D, Chairman. 1981a. *Obstacles, Report of the Special Committee on the Disabled and the Handicapped.* Ottawa: Ministry of Supply and Services, Canada.

Smith R. 1981b. Alcohol and alcoholism, the relation between consumption and damage. *British Medical Journal* 283:895–898.

Smith R. 1981c. Preventing alcohol problems, a job for Canute? *British Medical Journal* 283:972–975.

Snow J. 1936. *Snow on Cholera.* New York: The Commonwealth Fund.

Soltero I, Liu K, Cooper R, Stamler J, and Garside D. 1978. Trends in mortality from cerebrovascular diseases in the United States, 1960–1975. *Stroke* 9(6):549–555.

Sox HC. 1979. Quality of patient care by nurse practitioners and physician's assistants, a ten-year perspective. *Annals of Internal Medicine* 91:459–468.

Spitzer WO, Sackett DL, Sibley JC, et al. 1974. The Burlington randomized trial of the nurse practitioner. *New England Journal of Medicine* 290:251–256.

Stallones RA. 1980. The rise and fall of ischemic heart disease. *Scientific American* 243(5):53–59.

Stamler J. 1978. George Lyman Duff Memorial Lecture. Lifestyles, major risk factors, proof and public policy. *Circulation* 58(1):3–19.

Stamler J. 1979. Research related to risk factors. *Circulation* 60(7):1575–1587.

Stamler J. 1981. Disease of the cardiovascular system. In *Preventive and Community Medicine*, Second Edition, DW Clark and B MacMahon, eds., pp. 193–217. Boston: Little Brown and Company.

Stamler R, Stamler J, Lindberg HA, et al. 1979. Asymptomatic hyperglycaemia and coronary heart disease in middle-aged men in two employed populations in Chicago. *Journal of Chronic Diseases* 38:805–815.

Statistics Canada. 1981a. *Vital Statistics*, Vol. 1, Births and deaths, 1981. Catalogue 84–204. Annual. Ottawa: Ministry of Supply and Services, Canada.

Statistics Canada. 1981b. *The Health of Canadians, Report of the Canadian Health Survey.* Catalogue 82–538 E. Ottawa: Health and Welfare, Canada.

Statistics Canada. 1982a. *Vital Statistics*, Vol. 3, Mortality summary list of causes, 1980. Catalogue 84–206. Annual. Ottawa: Ministry of Supply and Services, Canada.

Statistics Canada.1982b. *Vital Statistics*, Vol. 1, Births and deaths, 1980. Catalogue 84–204. Annual. Ottawa: Ministry of Supply and Services, Canada.

Statistics Canada. 1983a. Cancer in Canada, 1979. Catalogue 82–207. Ottawa: Ministry of Supply and Services, Canada.

Statistics Canada. 1983b. *Statistics Canada Daily,* Tuesday February 1st, 1983. Ottawa: Federal and Media Relations Division.

Statistics Canada. 1985. *Vital Statistics, Vol. 1, Births and deaths, 1983.* Catalogue 84–204. Annual. Ottawa: Ministry of Supply and Services, Canada.

Steinfeld E, Schroeder S, Bishop M, Aiello J, Andrades S, and Buchanan R. 1976. Human factors research on building standards for accessibility to disabled people. In *The Behavioral Basis of Design*, Book 1, P Suedfeld and

JA Russell, eds., pp. 308–315. Stroudsburg, Pennsylvania: Dowden Hutchinson and Ross.

Szmuness W, Stevens CE, Harley EJ, et al. 1980. Hepatitis B vaccine. *New England Journal of Medicine* 303(15):833–841.

Task Force on Hypertension. 1978. *Final Report.* Toronto: Ontario Council of Health.

Thomas JE. 1983. *Medical Ethics and Human Life.* Toronto: Samuel Stevens.

Thomas L. 1978. Biomedical science and human health. *Yale Journal of Biology and Medicine* 51(2):133–142.

Townsend P, and Davidson N. eds. 1982. *Inequalities in Health, The Black Report.* Middlesex: Penguin Books.

Trinca GW, and Dooley BJ. 1975. The effects of mandatory seat belt wearing on the mortality and pattern of injury of car occupants involved in motor vehicle crashes in Victoria. *Medical Journal of Australia:* 675–678.

Trinca JC, ed. 1979. *Commonwealth Serum Laboratories Medical Handbook,* 1979 Edition. Parkville, Victoria: Commonwealth Serum Laboratories.

Tuyns AJ, Pequignot G, and Jensen OM. 1977. Le cancer de l'oesophage en Ille-et-Vilaine en fonction des niveaux de consommation d'alcool et de tabac. *Bulletin du Cancer* 64(1):45–60.

Ulrich RS. 1979. Visual landscapes and psychological well-being. *Landscape Research* 4(1):17–23.

United States Bureau of the Census. 1975. *Historical Statistics of the United States, Colonial Times to 1970.* Bicentennial Edition, Part 1. Washington, D.C.: U.S. Government Printing Office.

Vedin A, Wilhelmsson C, Tibblin G, and Wilhelmsen L. 1976. The post-infarction clinic in Goteborg, Sweden, A controlled trial of a therapeutic organization. *Acta Medica Scandinavica* 200:453–456.

Veterans Administration Cooperative Study Group on Antihypertensive Agents. 1967. Effects of treatment on morbidity in hypertension, 1, Results in patients with diastolic blood pressure averaging 115 through 129 mm Hg. *Journal of The American Medical Association* 202:1028–1034.

Veterans Administration Cooperative Study Group on Antihypertensive Agents. 1970. Effects of treatment on morbidity in hypertension, 2, Results in patients with diastolic blood pressure averaging 90 through 114 mm Hg. *Journal of the American Medical Association* 213:1143–1152.

Volk WA, and Wheeler MF. 1984. Basic microbiology (5th edition) (pp. 8, 266–267). New York: Harper and Row.

Wald N, Doll R, and Copeland G. 1981. Trends in tar, nicotine and carbon monoxide yields of U.K. cigarettes manufactured since 1934. *British Medical Journal* 282:763–765.

Wald N, Idle M, Boreham J and Bailey A. 1980. Low serum-vitamin-A and subsequent risk of cancer. Preliminary results of a prospective study. *Lancet* 2(8199):813–815.

Walker WJ. 1977. Editorial. Changing United States life-style and declining vascular mortality: cause or coincidence? *New England Journal of Medicine* 297(3):163–165.

White KL, Williams TF, and Greenberg BG. 1961. The ecology of medical care. *New England Journal of Medicine* 265(18):885–892.

White NF. 1981. Modern health concepts. In *The Health Conundrum*, NF White, ed., pp. 5–18. Toronto: TV Ontario Publications.

Wigle DT, and Mao Y. 1980. *Mortality by Income Level in Urban Canada.* Ottawa: Health and Welfare, Canada, Health Protection Branch.

Wilkins R. 1980a. *Health Status in Canada, 1926–1976.* Occasional Paper No. 13. Montreal: Institute for Research on Public Policy.

Wilkins R. 1980b. *Differential Mortality in Montreal, 1961–1976.* Paper Presented at the Annual Meeting of the Canadian Population Society, 6 June 1980, at Montreal.

Wilkins R, and Adams OB. 1982. *Health Expectancy in Canada, Late 70's, Demographic, Regional, and Social Dimensions.* Paper Read at Annual American Public Health Association Meeting, Population and Family Planning Section, November 1982, Montreal.

Wilner DM, Walkley RP, Pinkerton TC, et al. 1962. *The Housing Environment and Family Life.* Baltimore: Johns Hopkins University Press.

Wilson P. 1980. Drinking habits in The United Kingdom. *Population Trends* 1980(22):14–18.

Wissler RW. 1978. Current status of regression studies. In *Atherosclerosis Reviews 3*, R Paoletti and AM Gotto Jr., eds., pp. 213–229. New York: Raven Press.

World Health Organization. 1979. *Controlling the Smoking Epidemic, Report of The WHO Expert Committee on Smoking Control.* Technical Report Series No. 636. Geneva.

World Health Organization. 1980. *International Classification of Impairments, Disabilities and Handicaps.* Geneva.

World Health Organization. 1984a. *WHO Constitution Basic Documents*, Thirty-Fourth Edition. Geneva.

World Health Organization. 1984b. *World Health Statistics Annual, 1984.* Geneva.

Wynder, E, Blackburn H, Lewis B, et al. 1979. Conference on the health effects of blood lipids, optimal distributions for populations, epidemiological section. *Preventive Medicine* 8:609–678.

Wynder EL, and Graham EA. 1950. Tobacco smoking as a possible etiologic factor in bronchogenic carcinoma, a study of six hundred and eighty-four proved cases. *Journal of the American Medical Association* 143:329–336.

Young NA. 1979b. Poliovirus. In *Principles and Practice of Infectious Diseases*, GL Mandell, RG Douglas, and JE Bennett, eds., pp. 1091–1103. New York: John Wiley & Sons.

Young TK. 1979a. Changing patterns of health and sickness among the Cree-Ojibwa of northwestern Ontario. *Medical Anthropology* 3(2):191–223.

Index

Accidents, 22–24, 36, 39, 45–46, 50,
    54, 56, 87, 93, 100–102
  home, 44
  motor vehicle, 24, 42, 53, 88, 91,
    144–148, 151, 187
Acculturation, heart disease and,
    121–122
Activity restriction, 4, 30–31, 44,
    47–48, 58–61
Affluence and health, 89 90, 125–126
Age-specific death rates, 17, 19–21,
    75
Air-borne disease, 65–71
Alameda County Study, 33–34, 122
Alcohol, and disease, 87–89, 113–114
Alcohol consumption reduction,
    142–144
American elderly, 42–44
American Heart Association, 132, 136
American National Cooperative Study
    Group, 161
American Veterans Administration
    Trial, 160 161
Analogy, 79
Analytic survey, study design, 77–78
Angina pectoris, 160–161
Antibiotic therapy, 68–69, 153
Anti-coronary Club Trial, 136, 137
Asbestos, 95–97, 99
Australian Therapeutic Trial, 159
Avoidable causes of cancer, 110–116

B-carotene, protective effect, 113
Bed rest and heart attacks, 7–8, 153
Behavioral Sciences, 160, 191–192
Bias, 77, 128–129, 188
Biologic sense, 79

Biological, wall, 35
  aspects of heart disease, 122–124
  evidence and cancer, 105–108
Black Americans, 45–47
Blind assessment, 80–81
Breast, cancer treatment, 154 155
  examination, 155
British Doctor's study of smoking,
    85–86
British National Health Service, 173,
    182, 185
Brontë family, 17
Burkitt, D.P., 90

Canada Health Survey, 25–26, 30, 31,
    43
Canadian Indian population, 49–51
Canadian poor, 51–57
Canadian Sickness Survey, 25
Cancer
  causation, 84–85, 88, 90, 91, 93–99,
    104–116
  frequency, 26–27, 42, 45–46, 54
  primary prevention, 130–135
  treatment, 154–157
Carcinogenesis, 106–107
Case-control, study design, 77–78
Case series, study design, 77–78
Cassell, J., 100
Causation, methods, 75–79
Causes of, disease, 82–126
Cholera, 51, 65, 67, 69–70
Cholesterol, heart disease and,
    118–120, 124
  reducing strategies, 135–139
Cholestyramine, 138–139
Chromosomal disorders, 82–83

Clinical disagreement, 164–165
Cohort, 17
  inception, 80
  study design, 76–78
Co-intervention, 129
Co-morbidity, 128
Comparative mortality figures, by
    income, 53–55
Compliance, 128
  with health care, 174–175
  hypertension and, 159–160
Comprehensive care, 170, 193
Confounding variable, 75, 81
Consequences of disease, 4, 58–60
Consistency, 79
Consumer-choice health plan,
    181–182
Contamination, 128
Conundrum of heart disease, 125
Coronary by-pass surgery, 160–161
Coronary care units, 153, 161–163,
    170
Cost–benefit analysis, 178
Cost–containment incentives, 180–182
Cost–effectiveness analysis, 177–178
Cost minimization, 177
Cost–utility analysis, 178
Crude death rate, 19

Demographic aspects of health,
    34–36, 42–45
Deoxyribonucleic acid (DNA),
    106–107, 115, 123
Depression, 31, 32
Determinants of health, 72–73
Diabetes mellitus, 90
  heart disease and, 117–118
Diagnostic, criteria, 129
  accuracy, 165–166
Diarrhoeal diseases, 65–67, 69–70
Diet, and disease, 89–90, 111–113,
    118–120
Dietary carcinogenesis
  effects on carcinogens, 112–113
  ingestion, 112
  overnutrition, 111
  production, 112
  promotion, 113
Diptheria, 65, 69–70
Disability, 4, 28–39, 43–44, 58–60
Disease frequency, 16–61

Disease and illness, 2–5
Disease-oriented perspective, 14, 186,
    197
  challenge to, 152
  era, 1
  patient's perspective and, 191–194
  reductionist view, 185
Distributive justice, 12
Doctor-patient relationship, 193
Doll, Sir Richard, 94, 110–116
Dose-response gradient, 79
Driver education, 145
Driving behavior, and accidents, 91
  promoting safe, 144–148
Duration of stay, 28–29

Effectiveness, definition, 128
  evaluation criteria for, 128–129
  of health care system, 169–176
  need for evaluation of, 190–191
Efficacy definition, 128
Efficiency, of health care, 176–182,
    190–191
Emotional Health, 5, 31–32
Enthoven, Alain, 181
Environmental factors, and disease,
    92–102
Epidemiologic sense, 79
Epidemiological evidence and cancer
    causation, 108–110
Epidemiology of disability, 189–190
Eskimos, see Inuit
Ethics, 11–13
European Coronary Surgery Study,
    161
Evaluation, see Effectiveness; Efficacy;
    Efficiency
Exercise, and health, 90–91
Experimental evidence, 76–77

False negative, and positive, 166
Fee-for-service, pre-paid care and, 179
Follow-up, complete, 80, 129
Food additives, and cancer, 114
Food-borne disease, 65, 67, 69–70
Food supply, and mortality, 70–73

Genetic diseases, 82–83
Geophysical factors, cancer and, 115
Group practice, 169–170

Handicap, 4, 58-60
  mobility, 4
  occupation, 4
  orientation, 4
  self-care, 4
  self-sufficiency, 4
  social, 4
Health, 1-5, 14
Health care system, 168-183
Health economics, 176-182
Health education, 132-136, 139-148
Health expectancy, 31
Health and health care, 184-188
Health insurance plan of New York,
  170
  trial of breast screening, 155
Health maintenance organization, 170,
  178-180
Health policy, 10-14, 188-191
Healthfulness, 28
Healthy behavior patterns, 89
Heart disease
  causation, 84-86, 90, 98, 116-124
  frequency, 42, 45-46, 50, 54
  primary prevention, 135-142
  treatment, 160-163
Helsinki Mental Hospital Study, 137
Heredity, and disease, 82-83, 117
High density lipoprotein cholesterol,
  124, 141
Hill, Sir Austin Bradford, 76, 154
Hispanic Americans (Mexican, Cuban,
  Puerto Rican), 47-49
Hospital utilization, 29, 43, 48, 56
Hyperglycaemia, 117-118
Hypertension
  frequency, 43, 46
  heart disease and, 117
  treatment, 157-160, 175
Hypertension Detection and Follow-
  up Program, 159

Illness, see Consequences; Disability;
  Health; Morbidity
Immunization, 148-150
Impairment, 4, 58-60
Inception cohort, 80
Inclusion criteria, 128
Income, see Canadian poor
Indices of health, 16-61

Individuals who stop smoking,
  131-132
Industrial products, cancer and, 114
Industrialization and mortality, 67-72
Inequalities in health, 5
  black Americans, 45-47
  Canadian natives, 49-51
  Canadian poor, 51-57
  elderly, 42-45
  Hispanic Americans, 47-49
Infant diseases, and decline in
  mortality, 71
Infant mortality, 21, 24, 35, 71, 134
  black Americans, 45
  Canadian natives, 49
  Canadian poor, 53-54
Infanticide, 71
Infection, cancer and, 115-116
Infectious disease and decline in
  mortality, 35, 63-73
Initiation in carcinogenesis, 107, 116
Institutionalization, 29-30
International Atherosclerosis Project,
  119
International Classification of
  Impairments Disabilities and
  Handicaps, 58
Inuit, 49-51
Ionizing radiation, 115

Koch, Robert, 7, 76, 185
  postulates, 7

Legislation and driving behavior,
  146-148
  drunk driving, 147
  package of measures, 147-148
  seat-belt usage, 146-147
Life expectancy, 18, 34-35
  black Americans, 45
  Canadian Indians, 49
  methodology, 17
  rare extremes of, 35-36
  17th century, 41
  unequal changes, 41
Life span, 17, 35-36
Life-style, and disease, 84-92; see also
  specific behaviors
Lipid Research Clinics Trial, 138,
  139

Los Angeles Veterans Administration
    Trial, 137
Low density lipoprotein cholesterol,
    124, 138, 139, 141
Lung cancer, see Cancer, Smoking
    and disease

Mammography, and breast cancer,
    155
Man-made environment, 99-102
Maneuver, description of, 128
Mao, Y., 52
McClure, Walter, 181
McKeown, Thomas, 62-73, 152, 172
Measles, 65, 69-70
Medical education, 191-192
Medical research
    focus of, 1
    organization of care and, 175
Medical Research Council Trials, 149
Medical therapy, 152-163, 187
    evaluation methodology, 163-166
Medicines and medical procedures,
    cancer and, 115
Migration, and heart disease, 119,
    120, 122
    and cancer, 109
Molecular interactions, atherosclerosis
    and, 124
Morbidity
    frequency, 25-39
    health care and, 187-188
    subjectivity of, 193
Morris, J.N., 90
Mortality, 18, 21-25, 34-36
    cancer, 23-24, 155-157
    heart disease, 23-24, 162
    historical analysis, 62-73
    hygiene and, 70
    J-shaped curve, 22
    methodology, 19-21
    number of doctors and, 172
    peri-, neo-, postneonatal, 24-25
    premature, 35; See also specific
        populations
Multiple Risk Factor Intervention
    Trial, 134, 140-141
Multiple risk factor reduction,
    139-141
    MRFIT, 140-141
    Oslo Trial, 139-140

Multiple sclerosis, 59-60
Myocardial infarction, 160-163

National Ambulatory Medical Care
    Survey, 37-39
National Health Interview Survey,
    25-26, 30, 47
Natural history, of disease, 27, 73-81
Negative predictive value, 166
Ni-Hon-San Study, 122
Nonanalytic survey, study design,
    77-78
Non-infectious disease, and decline in
    mortality, 63-67, 71-73
Nurse practitioners, quality of care,
    171
Nutrition, and mortality, 70-73

Obesity, see Overeating
Occupational environment, and
    disease, 93-97, 114
Organizational structure of health
    care, 169-172
    specialization and, 192
Oslo Study, 134, 139-140
Outcomes, accuracy of, 80
    assessment of, 129
Overeating and disease, 89-90,
    111-112, 121

Patients
    allied health professions and, 193
    nurses' role and, 193
    perspective of, 3, 191-194
    responsiveness to, 193
    their role in medical education,
        192
Perinatal death rate, 24-25
Peto, Richard, 94, 110-116
Physically handicapped, 58-59
Platelets, atherosclerosis and, 123-124
Political process, 13-14
Pollution, and disease, 97-99, 114
Polycyclic hydrocarbons, and disease,
    95, 97, 99, 112
Pooling Project Research Group,
    117-118, 120
Population
    age structure, 34-36

concept of, 5-6
growth, 63
Population health
concepts, 2-6
definition, 1-2
perspective, 194-198
practice, 10-14
scientific basis of, 6-10
Population perspective on health,
194-198
an anthropological perspective, 196
distributive justice, 197
holism, 197-198
integration and, 194-195
a national health policy, 195
a numerical view, 196
Positive predictive value, 166
Pott, Percivall, 93
Predictive value, 165-166
Pre-paid medical service, see Health
maintenance organization
Primary care, integration, 191-193
morbidity in, 36-39
Primary prevention, 127-151,
186 187
by diet and cholesterol reduction,
135-139
immunization and, 148-150
interventions, 129-150
methods, 127-129
by multiple risk factor reduction,
139-142
to promote safe driving, 144-148
to reduce alcohol consumption,
142-144
of tobacco related disease, 130-135
Professional autonomy, 13
Prognosis, methods, 75-76, 79-81
Prognostic
factors adjustment, 81
stratification, 128
Promotion in carcinogenesis, 107,
113, 116
Promotion of safe driving, 144-148
Prostaglandin, 123
Protective factors, and effects of
smoking, 131
Psychosocial factors
heart disease and, 121-122

Quality of care
organizational determinants,
171-172
process measures, 173
Quality of life, 2-5
and alcohol, 88
and health care, 187-188
see also Morbidity

Random allocation, 128
Randomized controlled trial,
definition and importance of,
76-78
Referral pattern, 80
Relative odds, 78
Relative risk, 78
Reproductive and sexual behavior,
and disease, 91, 114
Respiratory disease, 23-24, 26-27,
37-39, 42, 46
Canadian natives, 50
Canadian poor, 54-56
in 19th century, 65-66, 68-70
and occupation, 94 97
and pollution, 98-99
and smoking, 84-85, 110-111,
130-131
Response to injury, hypothesis in
atherosclerosis, 123
Risk, of disease and illness, 62-125
definition, 73-75
factors, 9, 84-92, 110-122
methods, 75-79
Royal College of Physicians
guidelines to reduce exposure to
smoke, 132

Safe cigarette, 130-131
Scarlet fever, in 19th century, 65,
68-70
Screening, 163-164
for breast cancer, 154-155
for cervical cancer, 155-157
for hypertension, 158
Seat-belt usage, 145-148
Sensitivity, 165-166
Seven Countries Study, 117, 118,
119
Sewage disposal, 70

Single-gene disorders, 82
Smallpox in 19th century, 65–66, 69–70
Smoking, and disease, 12, 84–87
    and cancer, 110–111
    and heart disease, 118
    preventive strategies, 130–135, 139–141
Smoking cessation, 131–135
Snow John, 51
Social class, see Canadian poor
Social health, 5, 33–34, 92
    Alameda county, 33–34
Social network index, 34
Social relationships, and mortality, 92
Specificity
    of an association, 79
    of diagnostic test, 165–166
Standardization of death rates, 20–21
Standardized mortality ratio, 20–21
Stanford Heart Disease Prevention Program, 136
Starvation, 71, 89
Stepped care, hypertension, 159
Strength of association, 77–78
Stroke, 22–25, 29, 158
    black Americans, 45–46
    elderly, 42
Subpopulations, 5–6
Suicide, 23, 42–43, 46, 50, 51
Sulphur oxides, and disease, 98–99
Survival curve, 35–36
    rectangularization, 35–36
Synthetic chemicals, and cancer, 93, 114–115

Teeside Coronary Survey, 161–162
Temporality, 74, 79

Therapeutic interventions
    evaluation, 7–10, 128–129
Thrombosis, atherosclerosis and, 124
Tobacco, see Smoking
Tuberculosis, 11, 17, 35, 55, 65–66, 68–70
Two by two table, 76–78
Type A behavior, heart disease and, 121–122

United Airlines Trial, 137, 138
U.S. Veterans Study of Smoking, 84–85, 118
User fee, 181

Vaccination, 148–150
    BCG, 68
    declining mortality and, 67–73
    smallpox, 69
Vessel wall, atherosclerosis and, 123
Veterans Administration Cooperative Study, 158–159
Vitamin A, carcinogenesis and, 113
    cancer protection and, 131
Vitamin C, carcinogenesis and, 112

Water-borne disease, 65–67, 69–70
Water purification, 70
Well-being, 2–3
Western Collaborative Group Study, 121
WHO Cooperative Trial (clofibrate), 136, 137
Whooping cough, 65, 69–70
Wigle DT, 52
World Health Organization, 4, 58

Zero-time shift, 27, 164